HOW TO FIGHT MUSCLE LOSS AS YOU AGE? (SARCOPENIA)

Patrick Quan

SLICE OF LIFE MEDIA GROUP

Copyright © [2021] by [Patrick Quan]

All rights reserved.

No portion of this book may be reproduced in any form without written permission from the publisher or author, except as permitted by U.S. copyright law.

CONTENTS

Check out our other books — 4

Message Review for RockStar!! — 5

This book is dedicated — 6

SARCOPENIA — 7

PREFACE — 8

TABLE OF CONTENTS — 10

INTRODUCTION — 14

CHAPTER ONE — 17

CHAPTER TWO — 30

CHAPTER THREE — 41

CHAPTER FOUR — 49

CHAPTER FIVE — 54

CHAPTER SIX — 64

CHAPTER SEVEN — 69

CHAPTER EIGHT	74
CHAPTER NINE	94
CHAPTER TEN	101
CHAPTER ELEVEN	106
CHAPTER TWELVE	119
CHAPTER THIRTEEN	132
CONCLUSION	138
REFERENCES	142
THANK YOU	156

Check out our other books
Scan the QRcode below

Please click link below to check out other books

https://www.amazon.com/stores/author/B08PFF716J/allbooks?

Copyright © 2021 by Patrick Quan
SLICE OF LIFE MEDIA GROUP
ALL RIGHTS RESERVED

No part of this book may be reproduced
or used in any manner without written permission
of the copyright owner except for the
use of quotations in a book review.

For more information.
Email Address: info@sliceoflife.co

FIRST EDITION VOLUME 1

MESSAGE REVIEW FOR ROCKSTAR!!

Hello *RockStar!!*

Can I ask for a favor?

If you enjoyed this book, please take 3 mins to post your honest review on Amazon. It doesn't have to be elaborate: Just share your thoughts about the book, whether it helped you or not, and if so how & stuff like that.

Scan the QRcode below to review:

If you enjoyed this book, please consider dropping us a review on the link below:

https://www.amazon.com/review/create-review/?asin=B096TRWYWC

Support Small businesses like ours:
Every review helps & Your opinion matters!!
Please drop an email if you have any suggestions.
Email Address: info@sliceoflife.co

FIRST EDITION VOLUME 1

THIS : OOK IS DEDICATED

To my loving parents:

"Sir" Moon Pin Literati &
"Lady" Linda Ling Ho Quan
for nurturing and believing in me.
To my siblings and family for their support.
To my readers, I offer this book in service
to finding your inner self.
Find balance and tranquility, and become the best version of yourself.
Love.
Patrick Quan

SARCOPENIA

H OW TO FIGHT MUSCLE LOSS AS YOU AGE?

PREFACE

Sarcopenia plays a crucial role in maintaining your independence and quality of life as you age. How you manage your muscle mass directly impacts your mobility, strength, and overall health. The techniques behind fighting sarcopenia highlight the significance of taking action now and provide the tools to preserve your vitality.

"Aging is not lost youth but a new stage of opportunity and strength." - Betty Friedan

As you enter your middle age and beyond, you may notice changes in your body that seem inevitable. Your muscles may feel weaker, and everyday tasks become more challenging.

You might even resign yourself to the idea that this is just a normal part of aging.

But what if it didn't have to be this way?

Recent cutting-edge research has revealed that sarcopenia, the age-related loss of muscle mass and strength, is not an inevitable consequence of growing older. In fact, with the right strategies, you can maintain and even rebuild your muscles well into your golden years.

For decades, the prevailing advice for combating muscle loss has been to simply eat more protein and lift weights. While these are important components, they are not the whole picture.

Sarcopenia is a complex condition influenced by a variety of factors, from hormonal changes to inflammation and even your gut health. It is a condition characterized by loss of skeletal muscle mass and function. Although it is primarily a disease of the elderly, its development may be associated with conditions that are not exclusively seen in older persons.

Sarcopenia is a syndrome characterized by progressive and generalized loss of skeletal muscle mass and strength and it is strictly correlated with a physical disability, poor quality of life, and death. Risk factors for sarcopenia include age, gender, and level of physical activity. In conditions such as malignancy, rheumatoid arthritis, and aging, lean body mass is lost while fat mass may be preserved or even increased.

The loss in muscle mass may be associated with increased body fat so that despite normal weight there is marked weakness, this is a condition called sarcopenic obesity. There is an important correlation between inactivity and losses of muscle mass and strength, this suggests that physical activity should be a protective factor for the prevention but also the management of sarcopenia.

Furthermore, one of the first steps to be taken for a person with sarcopenia or clinical frailty is to ensure that the sarcopenic patient is receiving correct and sufficient nutrition. Sarcopenia has a greater effect on survival.

Here, we'll explore the cutting-edge science behind sarcopenia and reveal the little-known secrets to preserving your muscle mass. You'll explore why conventional wisdom has failed so many people and learn the surprising truth about what really works.

It should be important to prevent or postpone as much as possible the onset of this condition, to enhance survival, and to reduce the demand for long- term care. Interventions for sarcopenia need to be developed with the most attention on exercise and nutritional interventions.

Did you know that certain foods can actually accelerate muscle loss, even if they're high in protein? Or that the timing of your meals can be just as important as what you eat?

These are just a few of the revelations you'll encounter in the coming chapters.

You'll learn the three key pillars of muscle preservation and how to optimize each one for maximum results. You'll also explore the little-known supplements that can supercharge your efforts and the simple lifestyle changes that can make a profound difference.

Perhaps most importantly, you'll gain the knowledge and confidence to take control of your health and defy the stereotypes of aging. You'll see that sarcopenia is not a fate to be accepted but a challenge to be overcome.

TABLE OF CONTENTS

INTRODUCTION
CHAPTER ONE
What Is Sarcopenia

Sarcopenia

Is a Condition Known as Muscle Loss

Risk Factors

Histopathology

Sarcopenia

Management

Physiotherapy

CHAPTER TWO
The Effects of Sarcopenia and How to Fight It

How does Sarcopenia develop

Detrimental Effects of Sarcopenia

Can we Increase muscle mass as we get older

Stopping Sarcopenia before it starts

CHAPTER THREE
How to Tell If You Have Sarcopenia
How To Manage The Symptoms
What Can I Do To Manage Sarcopenia
Sarcopenia Treatment Supplements
Other nutritional supplements

CHAPTER FOUR
Aging and Why Do We Age
Global Aging Trends and
How Do They Affect Societies
Effects of Aging

CHAPTER FIVE
Sarcopenia - consequences
Effects of Endocrine Changes on Muscle
Gender differences
Is there a role for supplements

CHAPTER SIX
Causes of Sarcopenia

CHAPTER SEVEN
The Biological Mechanism of Sarcopenia
Factors That Contribute To Sarcopenia

CHAPTER EIGHT
How Can We Prevent Sarcopenia
Treatment Tips
What to Try First
Ways To Prevent Muscle Degeneration
Management Of Sarcopenia
How to Tell if You Are Losing Muscle Mass Due to Aging
How to Fight Sarcopenia and Muscle Wasting (Evidence-Based)

Exercise

Food and Nutrition to Help Prevent Muscle Deterioration

Other Ways to Help Prevent Sarcopenia

CHAPTER NINE

How to Fight Sarcopenia with Supplements

Why Supplements for Building Muscle Mass and Strength

CHAPTER TEN

Sarcopenia Treatment

CHAPTER ELEVEN

How to Fight Sarcopenia with Exercise

Exercise can help prevent sarcopenia

Types of Sarcopenia Exercises

Effect Of Exercise On Sarcopenia

Exercise Can Reverse Sarcopenia

Easy Exercises That Fight Muscle Loss as You Age

Tips To Fight Sarcopenia Through Proper Exercise And Nutrition

CHAPTER TWELVE

Nutrition's Role in Sarcopenia

Sarcopenia Stats

Nutrition Screening

Nutrition Care Process

Key Nutrition Recommendations

Protein

Vitamin D

Clinical Strategy

Physical Activity

Hormone and Drug Therapies

Prevention Is Key

CHAPTER THIRTEEN

What is good for Sarcopenia

HOW TO FIGHT MUSCLE LOSS AS YOU AGE? 13

Does Sarcopenia kill? How long patients do live
What should Sarcopenia Patients eat
Suggestions to Sarcopenia Patients
Strategies to Prevent Age-Related Muscle Loss
Start with an Understanding of Causes
Diagnosing Sarcopenia
CONCLUSION
REFERENCES
THANK YOU

INTRODUCTION

Sarcopenia is the loss of muscle mass that happens to everyone with age. However, the rate of sarcopenia and the severity of its sequelae vary greatly according to health status, physical activity, and possibly diet. In this book, I will discuss How to fight muscle loss as you age. (Sarcopenia) Symptoms, Causes, Treatment, Prevention, Exercise, Supplements, Food Nutrients, Diet and potential mechanisms of sarcopenia and some tips and ideas about prevention and treatment.

The term sarcopenia was initially used by Rosenberg to describe the loss of lean body mass with aging. For several years, it was used by scientists to refer only to the loss of skeletal muscle mass. More recently, in 2010, the European Working Group on Sarcopenia in Older People (EWGSOP) expanded the definition to include the presence of impaired performance measured by walking speed and/or muscle weakness in handgrip strength testing and proposed an algorithm for a systematic evaluation of persons with possible sarcopenia. This first consensus represented a significant development because it went beyond the static evaluation of muscle mass and underscored the physiologic and functional consequences of muscle atrophy with advanced adult age. In fact, from a functional and rehabilitative perspective, the addition of walking speed makes sense because this measurement correlates very well with the prevalence of limitations in activities of daily living, mobility, and survival. It has been reported that in many countries around the world, the prevalence of limitations in activities of daily living is higher in older age groups.

The proposal by the EWGSOP was followed by similar efforts by the International Working Group on Sarcopenia, the American Foundation for the National Institutes of Health, and the Asian Working Group on Sarcopenia (AWGS). The latter group updated their criteria in a more recent publication. There are some differences among these proposals but many more similarities and agreement.

Worldwide advances in applied science and health care technology, along with socio-economic development, have increase lifespan. In 2019, it was estimated that globally 703 million people were older than 65 years old and that this number would reach 1.5 billion by 2050. All nations have seen an increase in life expectancy with a disproportionately greater increase in elderly populations. Consequently, healthcare services are strained under the additional burden of increasing elderly populations. A better understanding of age-related chronic diseases and new modalities are required to address aging-related diseases and alleviate pressure on healthcare systems. One such disease is sarcopenia.

Sarcopenia is the progressive and generalized loss of muscle mass and function (i.e., strength) that occurs with age and is strongly associated with frailty. Frailty is defined by the vulnerability of the elderly to possible stressors that increase the risk for poor health outcomes, incident disability, and mortality.

Recent studies have revealed that sarcopenia is not a simple condition caused by nutrient deficiency or a sedentary lifestyle, but a result of elaborate multi- pathway pathogenesis.

From the time you are born to around the time you turn 30, your muscles grow larger and stronger. But at some point in your 30s, you start to lose muscle mass and function. This cause is age-related sarcopenia or sarcopenia with aging.

Physically inactive people can lose as much as 3% to 5% of their muscle mass each decade after age 30. Even if you are active, you'll still have some muscle loss. There's no test or specific level of muscle mass that will diagnose sarcopenia. Any loss of muscle matters because it lessens strength and mobility. Sarcopenia typically happens faster around age 75. But it may also speed up as early as 65 or as late as 80. It's a factor in frailty and the likelihood of falls and fractures in older adults.

CHAPTER ONE

What Is Sarcopenia

Sarcopenia is defined as being a decline in muscle function (either walking speed or grip strength) associated with loss of muscle mass. Sarcopenia most commonly affects elderly and sedentary populations and patients who have comorbidities that affect the musculoskeletal system or impair physical activity. Sarcopenia leads to disability, falls, and increased mortality. Loss of muscle strength and aerobic function is 2 of the hallmarks of frailty. Sarcopenia has been linked to an increased prevalence of osteoporosis, thus further increasing its propensity to produce fractures. Sarcopenia is a growing global health concern.

- Sarcopenia has been reported to affect 5-13% of persons aged 60 to 70 years and up to 50% of people over 80 years of age.

- In 2000, the number of people ≥ 60 years old around the world was estimated to be 600 million.

- This population is expected to rise to 1.2 billion by 2025 and 2 billion by 2050.

- Even with a conservative estimate of prevalence, sarcopenia affects >50 million people today and will affect >200 million in the next 40 years.

- Strength training should be considered a first-line treatment strategy for managing and preventing sarcopenia

Sarcopenia literally means "lack of flesh." It's a condition of age-associated muscle degeneration that becomes more common in people over the age of 50. After middle age, adults lose 3% of their muscle strength every year, on average. This limits their ability to perform many routine activities.

Unfortunately, sarcopenia also shortens life expectancy in those it affects, compared to individuals with normal muscle strength.

Sarcopenia is caused by an imbalance between signals for muscle cell growth and signals for teardown. Cell growth processes are called "anabolism," and cell teardown processes are called "catabolism".

For example, growth hormones act with protein-destroying enzymes to keep muscle steady through a cycle of growth, stress or injury, destruction, and then healing. This cycle is always occurring, and when things are in balance, muscle keeps its strength over time.

However, during aging, the body becomes resistant to the normal growth signals, tipping the balance toward catabolism and muscle loss. Your body normally keeps signals for growth and teardown in balance. As you age, your body becomes resistant to growth signals, resulting in muscle loss.

Sarcopenia is a type of muscle loss (muscle atrophy) that occurs with aging and/or immobility. It is characterized by the degenerative loss of skeletal muscle mass, quality, and strength. The rate of muscle loss is dependent on exercise level, co-morbidities, nutrition, and other factors. The muscle loss is related to changes in muscle synthesis signaling pathways. It is distinct from cachexia, in which muscle is degraded through cytokine-mediated degradation, although both conditions may co-exist. Sarcopenia is considered a component of frailty syndrome. Sarcopenia can lead to reduced quality of life and disability.

Sarcopenia is a factor in changing body composition associated with aging populations. In population studies, body mass index (BMI) is seen to decrease in aging populations while bioelectrical impedance analysis (BIA) shows body fat proportion rising.

The term sarcopenia is from Greek σάρξ sarx, "flesh" and πενία penia, "poverty". This was first proposed by Rosenberg in 1989, who wrote that "there may be no single feature of age-related decline that could more dramatically affect ambulation, mobility, calorie intake, and overall nutrient intake and status, independence, breathing, etc. Why have we not given it more attention? Perhaps it needs a name derived from the Greek. I'll suggest a couple: *sarcomalacia or sarcopenia*". As we get older our bodies naturally change in many ways, including muscle strength. But sometimes this goes beyond normal age-related processes and can become a health concern, including Sarcopenia. How can we prevent it from affecting our quality of life?

Sarcopenia is a disorder characterized by a loss of muscle mass and muscle strength. It's associated with the natural aging process as well as geriatric medical conditions and bed-rest. Sarcopenia is a progressive disease that mainly affects individuals over the age of 50 – affecting balance, strength, and the overall ability to complete everyday activities. While Sarcopenia can decrease life expectancy, it primarily affects a person's overall quality of life, leading to:

- Falls and fractures

- Weight loss and/or malnutrition

- Physical disability

- Poor quality of life, Institutionalization

- Morbi-mortality

- Increased healthcare costs

Skeletal muscle size and function vary greatly at all ages and during normal aging skeletal muscle size and function decline. Skeletal muscle size, the number of muscle fibers per muscle (30), the size of muscle fibers, and muscle strength already vary at least 2-fold in young individuals. During aging muscles additionally become smaller, weaker, and slower. For example, 75-year-old women and men lose 0.64-0.70% and 0.80-0.98% of their muscle mass and 2.5- 3% and 3-4% of their strength per year, respectively. This phenomenon is defined as sarcopenia, based on the Greek words sarx for flesh and penia for loss.

Some researchers additionally define the age-associated loss of strength as dynapenia but this seems superfluous as broadly defined sarcopenia includes losses of muscle function. An important subtype of sarcopenia is sarcopenic obesity which is defined as the presence of both sarcopenia and obesity. A workable diagnosis criterion for sarcopenia is the combination of "low muscle mass" and "low muscle strength" or "low physical performance".

While specific diagnostic criteria for sarcopenia have been published there is still no commonly used, cheap, easy-to-administer diagnostic test to identify patients with sarcopenia.

Sarcopenia Is a Condition Known as Muscle Loss

It mostly affects people who have passed their fifties, and it can decrease life expectancy and quality. The peak muscle mass is usually achieved in the late 30s and early 40s when a gradual loss of muscle mass begins.

Sarcopenia can occur quicker than you may think as physically inactive people can lose as much as 3-5% of their muscle mass each decade after the age of 30. As there is a strong relationship between strength and muscle mass, any loss of muscle mass is a cause for concern, although there is no specific level of muscle mass or lean body mass at which someone can say sarcopenia is present. This condition can significantly contribute to a decrease in life quality.

Sarcopenia can't be prevented, but luckily, it can be slowed down when people enter their 30s.

Get your hormones in balance

Muscle mass can greatly be affected by hormonal factors. A hormonal imbalance can directly affect sarcopenia, for women in particular, as concentrations of the hormone estradiol get reduced during the menopause in middle-aged and older women. During the post-menopausal period, the production of ovarian hormones decreases, which leads to impaired muscle performance. As a hormonal imbalance and changes may play a significant role in sarcopenia in older women, it is advised to track hormone levels during an annual blood work. When it comes to men, they should check their testosterone, growth hormone, and DHEA levels, and try to bring their hormones in balance using natural supplementation.

Increase the intake of dietary protein

When it comes to building and repairing muscle fibers, protein is the most valuable food. People over age 70 tend to eat less than recommended (which is 0.8 g of protein per kg of body weight). However, adults who are 65 and older need higher levels of dietary protein, up to 1.2 g of protein per kg of body weight. This is a great target for daily protein intake for healthy adults. As for those with sarcopenia, their protein intake should be 1.5 g/kg of protein a day.

In order to know how much protein you need, take your body weight (in kilograms) and multiply it by 1.2, which will give you the recommended amount of protein per day. For example, if you weigh 70 kg, aim for about 85 g of protein per day. Fish, poultry, and most meat have 7 g of protein in an ounce, while one egg or one cup of milk can supplement you with 8 g of protein. Eat high-protein snacks between meals to reach your daily protein count.

Omega-3 fatty acids

According to a study published in 2011, omega-3 fatty acids may be useful for the treatment and prevention of sarcopenia as they are found to stimulate the synthesis of muscle protein in older adults. Omega-3 fatty acids have anti- inflammatory effects and help to preserve muscle mass under different physiological conditions. To increase your omega-3 acid intake, consider supplementing your diet with flaxseed oil or fish oil, or add salmon, herring, trout, white fish, tuna, chia seeds, walnuts, anchovies, and hemp seeds to your shopping list.

Walk

Walking is an activity that people can do anywhere, and it is known to prevent sarcopenia (and even reverse the process). Sarcopenia is best fought when you use your muscles and walking gives a workout to your glutes and tones your calves, hamstrings, and quadriceps. To avoid injury and prevent the process of sarcopenia, it is of the utmost importance to exercise every muscle group you can and prevent losing lean muscle mass.

Strength training

If you lead a sedentary lifestyle, you must give up on it as soon as possible because your muscles need to be active in order not to lose their mass. Equip yourself with some quality bodybuilding clothes that allow your body to breathe and move freely, and start with a strength training routine. Among other things, strength training includes pulling resistance bands and weightlifting. During strength training, your body strength gets increased due to tension on your muscle fibers and the increased action of hormones that promote growth. All of these cause muscle cells to repair themselves and grow – a process that directly affects the prevention of muscle mass loss.

Sarcopenia can be prevented or reversed even with simple exercises such as walking. Exercising is the most effective way of battling the condition, especially strength training. Go to your local gym and ask the staff to show you some strength training exercises, like lifting weights, calisthenics, and how to use resistance bands. Supplement yourself with enough protein and creatine, as well as omega-3 supplements, to increase your life quality and maintain healthy muscle mass.

Risk Factors

Sarcopenia is considered by most to be an inevitable part of aging. However, the degree of sarcopenia is highly variable and is dependent upon the presence of certain risk factors:

Physical Inactivity:

Lack of exercise is believed to be the foremost risk factor for sarcopenia. A gradual decline in myocyte numbers begins around 50 years of age. The decline in muscle fiber and strength is more pronounced in patients with a sedentary lifestyle as compared to patients who are physically more active. Even professional athletes such as marathon runners and weight lifters show a gradual (more slow) decline in their speed and strength with aging.

Hormone and Cytokine Imbalance:

Age-related decreases in hormone concentrations (eg testosterone, thyroid hormone, and insulin-like growth factor) lead to loss of muscle mass and

strength. Extreme muscle loss often results from a combination of diminishing hormonal anabolic signals and promotion of catabolic signals mediated through pro-inflammatory cytokines.

Protein Synthesis and Regeneration:

A decrease in the body's ability to synthesize protein, coupled with an inadequate intake of calories and/or protein to sustain muscle mass, is common in sarcopenia. Oxidized proteins increase in skeletal muscle with aging and lead to a buildup of lipofuscin (yellowish-brown, pigmented, insoluble granules).[5] The age-related increase in amounts of oxidized protein may reflect the age-dependent accumulation of unrepaired DNA damage that affects the concentrations or activities of numerous factors that govern the rates of protein oxidation and the degradation of oxidized protein[6]. This accumulation of non-contractile dysfunctional protein in skeletal muscles is part of the reason muscle strength decreases severely in sarcopenia.

Motor Unit Remodelling:

Age-related reduction in motor nerve cells responsible for sending signals from the brain to the muscles to initiate movement also occurs. Satellite cells are small mononuclear cells that abut muscle fibers and are normally activated upon injury or exercise. In response to these signals, satellite cells differentiate and fuse into the muscle fiber, helping to maintain muscle function. One current hypothesis is that sarcopenia is caused, in part, by a failure in satellite cell activation.

Histopathology

Early sarcopenia is characterized by a decrease in the size of muscle and muscle tissue. Changes include:

Replacement of muscle fibers with fat, an increase in fibrosis, changes in muscle metabolism, oxidative stress, and degeneration of the neuromuscular junction.

This ultimately leads to progressive loss of muscle function and to frailty.

Sarcopenia predominantly affects the type II (fast-twitch) muscle fibers, type I (slow-twitch) fibers are much less affected.

Sarcopenia represents both a reduction in muscle fiber number as well as reduced fiber size.

Histological studies comparing muscle cross-sections of the elderly with those of younger individuals reveal at least 50% fewer type I and type II fibers by the ninth decade.

Screening Tools to Identify Sarcopenia

The SARC-F (Strength, assistance with walking, rising from a chair, climbing stairs, and falls) questionnaire

Assessing sarcopenia: muscle strength

Handgrip test: Generally, handgrip strength is one of the two methods utilized to quantify muscle strength in patients with suspected sarcopenia. Handgrip strength correlates with strength in other muscles and is therefore used as a surrogate to detect deficits in overall strength.

Chair stand test: The chair stand test may be used as a proxy to gauge lower extremity strength, particularly the quadriceps muscles. Suggested tests for sarcopenia severity include:

- Gait Speed Test

- TUG

- Pharmacological Treatment

Currently, there are no agents for the treatment of sarcopenia that have been FDA approved.

DHEA and human growth hormone have little to no effect. Growth hormone increases muscle protein synthesis and increases muscle mass but does not lead to gains in strength and function.

Testosterone or other anabolic steroids have a modest positive effect on muscle strength and mass but are of limited use due to adverse effects, such as the increased risk of prostate cancer in men, virilization in women, and overall increased risk of cardiovascular events.

New therapies for sarcopenia are in clinical development. Selective androgen receptor modulators (SARMs) are of particular interest because of their tissue selectivity. Other compounds under investigation as treatments for sarcopenia include myostatin, vitamin D, angiotensin-converting enzyme inhibitors, omega-3 supplements, and anabolic agents such as ghrelin and its analogs.

Sarcopenia Management Physiotherapy

Early recognition and intervention are the keys to improved outcomes in patients with sarcopenia. Screening patients for impairment in their physical function and activities of daily living (ADLs) should be a routine part of healthcare visits for the elderly. Assessment of patients' environments for fall hazards and implementation of precautionary safety measures should be part of the treatment strategy. An exercise regimen is considered a cornerstone in the treatment of sarcopenia.

A well-designed, progressive resistance exercise training program is well known to exert positive effects on both the nervous and muscular systems and, ultimately, results in profound enhancements in muscle mass and muscle strength.

Strength exercise training should be considered a first-line treatment strategy for managing and preventing both sarcopenias.

Short-term resistance exercise has been demonstrated to increase the ability and capacity of skeletal muscle to synthesize proteins.

Both resistance training (RT) and strength training (ST) of muscles have been shown to be somewhat successful interventions in the prevention and treatment of sarcopenia. RT has been reported to positively influence the neuromuscular system as well as increase hormone concentrations and the rate of protein synthesis.

The greatest effects are observed when resistance training and high protein diets are combined and appear to act synergistically. Specifically, consuming 20-35 grams of protein per meal is advised, as such amounts provides sufficient amino acid content to maximize MPS, thus minimizing age-related muscle loss. eg

Chicken Breast: 23.1 g Protein Per 100 g,
Canned Tuna: 23.6 g Protein Per 100 g,
Cocoa: 20 g Protein Per 100 g,
Cheddar Cheese: 24.9 g Protein Per 100 gv
Beef Jerky: 33.2 g Protein Per 100 g.

Additionally, patients with sarcopenia are recommended to consume 1.0 - 1.2 g/kg (body weight)/day.

CHAPTER TWO

The Effects of Sarcopenia and How to Fight It

Sarcopenia is the age-related loss of skeletal muscle mass and function. The name is relatively new, having been coined in 1989, and it literally means loss of flesh. Creepy name notwithstanding, it's an important condition we all need to learn more about.

Sarcopenia can be understood by knowing its symptoms. They include decreased mobility, physical inactivity, slow gait speed, poor endurance, weakness, and early death. In fact, one meta-analysis of 3,797 people suggested an increased risk of mortality for individuals diagnosed with sarcopenia versus those without it.

While has been a lot of research on sarcopenia's effects there is currently no generally accepted clinical definition of it. Many work from the definition crafted by the European Working Group on Sarcopenia in Older People (EWGSOP) who, along with other groups, reached a consensus on what objective measures to use to diagnose sarcopenia:

- Presence of low skeletal muscle mass and low muscle strength or low muscle performance.

- Walking speed and grip strength are used to measure strength.

- Low is classified as muscle mass estimated to be two standard deviations.

Below a normal young person's average.

At first glance, sarcopenia may resemble what we assume will happen to us all as we age. However, it is a specific condition that affects 14% of people aged 65-70 and 53% of people above the age of 80. These percentages are significant, but sarcopenia is not inevitable if the right steps are taken.

How does Sarcopenia develop?

The problem is that as we age we lose muscle mass. Many of us are on track to lose 3% to 5% every decade after 30. In fact, most men will lose about 30% of their muscle mass during their lifetime. The causes for this are varied and include obesity, diabetes, inadequate nutrition, and a decline in hormone levels.

Testosterone is one of the hormones that naturally declines as we get older. It, along with human growth hormone, are key to stimulating protein synthesis and muscle growth. As their levels drop so does our ability to create new muscle mass. Though testosterone is thought of as a male hormone, the drop in its production occurs in women as well, creating the same dip in muscle production.

"As we get older we tend to be less involved in physical activities. Moving our bodies, however, is exactly how we create more muscle."

What you eat also plays a huge role in whether or not you'll show signs of sarcopenia. For one, eating healthy reduces the risk of obesity or diabetes, both key factors for sarcopenia. Secondly, our ability to synthesize protein diminishes with age. This is especially true for men, who experience a phenomenon called anabolic resistance when they get older. This lowers their bodies' ability to utilize the protein.

One of the most important factors in advancing sarcopenia is inactivity. As we get older we tend to be less involved in physical activities. Moving our bodies, however, is exactly how we create more muscle. This can create a cycle where inactivity leads to weakness, making it more difficult to be physically active. The resulting muscle loss leads to more inactivity, and so on.

These factors all contribute to the breakdown of muscle mass that, when left unchecked, can lead to sarcopenia. Facing these challenges head-on may seem daunting, but with the right plan in place overcoming these issues—at any age—is possible.

Detrimental Effects of Sarcopenia

Sarcopenia as a condition threatens the ability of an individual to live independently. Functional reserve can be slowly worn away with aging or drop suddenly with injury, illness, hospitalization, or institutionalization. Health care costs alone, calculated in dollar value from 2000, were estimated to total over $18.5 billion ($10.8 billion for men, $7.7 billion for women), which accounted for 1.5% of the total annual health care. This would cost sarcopenic men and women an extra $860 and $933 per year, respectively. Even a 10% reduction in prevalence of this modifiable economic burden would save $1.1 billion per year in U.S. healthcare costs. The risk of complications, such as infections, pressure ulcers, loss of autonomy, institutionalization, poor quality of life, as well as for mortality, are also higher for hospitalized patients with sarcopenia.

A loss of muscle mass will reduce the maximum volume of oxygen update (VO2max), but age-related decrease in mitochondrial protein and myosin heavy chain synthesis rates have also been observed, which may explain some of features of sarcopenia. Increased age is also associated with anabolic resistance, increased sedentary lifestyle, higher body fat, increases in inflammation, decrease in muscle quality (intramuscular fat infiltration) and poly-medication. The detrimental effects of age on muscle motor neurons may account for the loss in strength observed in older adults. Muscle is influenced by its environment which has many positive and negative inputs, for example low vitamin D status and inflammatory conditions diminish muscle but physical activity and protein intake stimulate muscle.

See Figure below for framework of the environmental impact on muscle tissue.

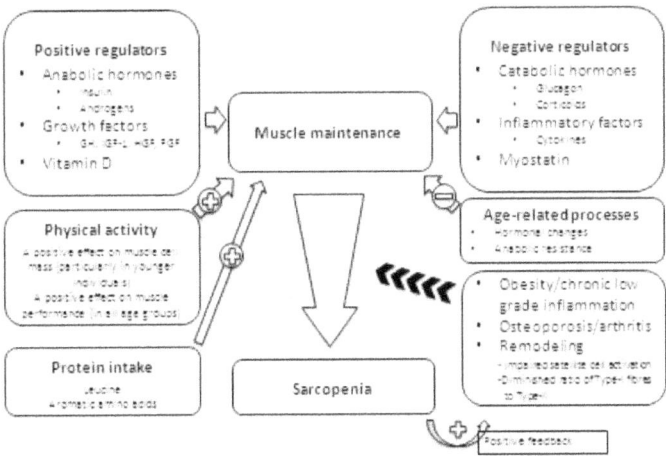

(Environmental factors affecting muscle tissue status)

Mobility disorders, increased risk of falls and fractures, impaired ability to perform activities of daily living, disabilities, loss of independence and increased risk of death are associated with the impaired health of a sarcopenic individual. The reduction in muscle mass and decrease in physical function which defines sarcopenia is associated with gradual decline in quality of life.

A four-year follow-up of community-dwelling men and women over 71 years of age or older showed that lower SPPB scores were associated with significant, gradual increase in the frequency of disability at follow-up, and after adjustment for age, sex and chronic disease those with the lowest scores were 4.2-4.9 times as likely to have disability at follow-up compared with those with the highest scores.

The physical functioning was predictive of likelihood of fractures, cognitive outcomes, cardiovascular disease, hospitalization and institutionalization in older community-dwelling populations. Over 1,000 men and women from age 20 to 102 years old observing considerable reduction in isometric muscle strength and muscle power with age, which was subsequently associated with poor mobility (gait speed less than 0.8m/s and inability to walk 1km).

Can we Increase muscle mass as we get older?

The causes of sarcopenia are many, but there are strategies that you can put in place to help you remain outside of that 14% of us that will develop sarcopenia as we move into our 60s.

Diet: Modifying your diet for long-term health is key to decreasing your risk of sarcopenia. With our body's ability to synthesize proteins reduced, we need to compensate by incorporating greater amounts of protein into our meals. Adding this extra protein into an overall better diet, balanced with quality carbs and fats, will also help boost the production of hormones that help build muscles, such as testosterone. Eating healthy improves your life in more ways than one. Add reducing the risk of sarcopenia to that list.

Sleep: To keep those hormones associated with muscle growth at healthy levels it's also important to combine a good diet with good sleep. In men, about 70% of the body's release of Human Growth Hormone happens as they sleep. This hormone stimulates muscle growth, while also strengthening bones and boosting heart health. As you get older, getting the proper amount of sleep becomes even more important.

Exercise: One of the most important and self-evident ways to produce more muscle is by exercising. Scientific studies reinforce this link and list regular physical activity as a protective factor in the prevention of sarcopenia. Although we tend to lose muscle mass as we get older, proper strength training exercises can push back against this trend, or even reverse it.

One study performed in 1994 backs this up by showing how a group of people were able to gain muscle mass even in their late 90s. This was done through a high-intensity, progressive regimen of resistance exercise training. The result was improved muscle strength and size, astonishingly, in individuals previously described as "frail" and "elderly."

Exercise also affects the connection between our brain and muscle fibers. The point of contact for this connection is called the neuromuscular junction and it's turned on whenever our muscles contract. When we work out we enhance this connection, allowing us to more effectively use our muscles to prevent or treat sarcopenia.

Stopping Sarcopenia before it starts

It's never too late to begin a plan that will help you fight sarcopenia. At the age of 80, the proper implementation of strength training exercises can still lead to muscle hypertrophy—an increase in the size of skeletal muscle—personal training with a kinesiologist makes preventing sarcopenia easy.

You may not realize it, but sarcopenia, the age-related loss of muscle mass and strength, can start as early as your 30s. By the time you reach your 50s, you could be losing up to 1% of your muscle mass each year. This gradual decline might seem insignificant at first, but over time, it can lead to frailty, increased risk of falls, and a loss of independence. The good news is that you can take steps to prevent sarcopenia before it even starts.

Think of your muscles as a powerful engine that propels you through life. Just like any engine, your muscles need regular maintenance and the right fuel to keep running smoothly. This is where a combination of proper nutrition and exercise comes into play.

First, let's talk about nutrition. Your muscles thrive on protein, the building block of life. To keep your muscles strong and healthy, you need to consume adequate amounts of high-quality protein. Aim for at least 0.8 grams of protein per kilogram of body weight daily, spread out across your meals. Good sources of protein include lean meats, fish, eggs, dairy products, beans, and nuts.

But protein alone isn't enough. Your muscles also need a balanced diet rich in fruits, vegetables, whole grains, and healthy fats to function optimally. These nutrients provide the vitamins, minerals, and antioxidants necessary to support muscle health and prevent inflammation, which can contribute to muscle loss. Now, let's talk about the other crucial component: exercise. Regular physical activity is essential for maintaining and even increasing muscle mass as you age.

Engage in a combination of resistance training and aerobic exercise to reap the most benefits. Resistance training, such as lifting weights or using resistance bands, challenges your muscles and stimulates growth. Aim for at least two to three strength training sessions per week, targeting all major muscle groups. Remember, it's never too late to start. Even if you've never lifted weights before, you can begin with simple exercises and gradually progress as you build strength and confidence.

The key to preventing sarcopenia is to adopt a proactive approach that combines a protein-rich diet with regular resistance training and aerobic exercise. Aerobic exercise, like brisk walking, swimming, or cycling, is also important for maintaining muscle health. It improves blood flow, delivering oxygen and nutrients to your muscles, and helps reduce inflammation.

Aim for at least 150 minutes of moderate-intensity aerobic activity per week.

In addition to nutrition and exercise, other lifestyle factors can impact muscle health. Getting enough sleep, managing stress, and avoiding smoking and excessive alcohol consumption can all contribute to the prevention of sarcopenia.

As the old saying goes, "An ounce of prevention is worth a pound of cure." By taking proactive steps to maintain your muscle mass and strength, you can stave off sarcopenia and enjoy a higher quality of life as you age.

CHAPTER THREE

How to Tell If You Have Sarcopenia

The signs of sarcopenia are the result of diminished muscle strength. Early signs of sarcopenia include feeling physically weaker over time and having more difficulty than usual lifting familiar objects.

A hand-grip-strength test has been used to help diagnose sarcopenia in studies and may be used in some clinics.

Decreased strength might show itself in other ways too, including walking more slowly, becoming exhausted more easily, and having less interest in being active.

Losing weight without trying can also be a sign of sarcopenia. However, these signs can also occur in other medical conditions. Yet if you experience one or more of these and can't explain why to talk to a health professional. Noticeable loss of strength or stamina and unintentional weight loss are signs of multiple diseases, including sarcopenia. If you are experiencing any of these without a good reason, talk to your doctor.

How To Manage The Symptoms

Sarcopenia can impact the quality of life and your ability to live independently as you age. It is seen as a normal part of the aging process affecting up to 10 percent of adults over the age of 50. If you have been diagnosed with sarcopenia, it's not too late to take steps toward treating and preventing further complications from sarcopenia.

Use this chapter to learn more about the best sarcopenia treatment options for you.

Sarcopenia is a muscular degenerative disorder common in older adults that means "lack of flesh." In a healthy person, growth hormones signal properly for growth and teardown of cells. An imbalance between this process causes sarcopenia.

Factors such as ;

- lack of exercise or movement

- diets low in calories and protein

- inflammation

- chronic illness

- severe stress are all contributors to sarcopenia.

Early signs of sarcopenia may not be visually noticeable, but you may feel weaker and have difficulty lifting. As it progresses, walking or using stairs may become harder and take more energy.

Loss of muscle mass and energy can be reversed or prevented if you take the proper steps as soon as possible.

What Can I Do To Manage Sarcopenia?

The best way to prevent further muscle loss due to sarcopenia is to begin an exercise routine. Resistance training is used most commonly to treat muscle loss in older patients in physical therapy programs. This type of exercise involves using dumbbells, exercise tubing or bands, and elliptical machines to build up your muscle strength and improve stamina.

Low-impact exercises like swimming, yoga, cycling, or even ballroom dancing are all good options to be more active without causing severe impact on your joints.

Other types of treatments that may work for sarcopenia include hormone replacement therapy or HRT. HRT has been shown to increase body mass, cut down on abdominal fat, and prevent osteoporosis in postmenopausal women. Other forms of treatment that may improve the symptoms of sarcopenia are testosterone supplements, vitamin D, and certain medications used to treat metabolic syndromes.

However, the risks associated with HRT do not make this the best option for treating sarcopenia. In conjunction with exercise, making sure you are getting proper nutrition is important to prevent further muscle desegregation and complications.

Sarcopenia Treatment Supplements

The essential supplement you need for treating sarcopenia is protein. It is essential for gaining and maintaining strength and improving mobility. The Mayo Clinic recommends people with, or at risk for sarcopenia should eat 1.2 to 1.5 grams of protein per kilogram of weight, or about 3.5-4.3 ounces for an adult who weighs 180 pounds.

To figure out how much protein you need, multiply 0.36 by your weight in pounds. Protein should comprise 15 to 25% of the calories you eat in a day. Your meals should contain 20 to 30 grams of protein in order to reach your daily recommended value.

If you need more protein to add to your diet, consider these foods that are great sources of protein:

Eggs: six grams of protein per serving

Almonds: six grams of protein per serving

Chicken breast: 53 grams of protein per serving

Oats: 11 grams of protein per serving

Cottage cheese: 28 grams of protein per serving

Greek yogurt: 17 grams of protein per serving

Milk: eight grams of protein per serving

Broccoli: three grams of protein per serving

Lean beef: 25 grams of protein per serving

Tuna: 27 grams of protein per serving

You do not have to get protein through food alone. If you have difficultly digesting food like beef or chicken breast, you can add protein to your diet in the form of nutritional supplements such as protein powders or capsules, and nutritional shakes.

Any dietary changes, like increasing your protein intake, should be done under the supervision of your doctor. Increasing your protein intake on your own is not recommended for people with impaired kidney function.

Other nutritional supplements

While protein-coupled with an exercise routine is very important for managing the symptoms of sarcopenia, other vitamins and mineral supplements may be helpful or even necessary. You may be lacking the proper nutrition in your diet to maintain bone and tissue health. These vitamins and minerals are essential for patients with sarcopenia:

Calcium

Calcium not only helps strengthen your bones, but it also plays an important role in muscle function. Calcium regulates the contraction and movement of your muscles. This is important for building up muscle strength.

A good source of this mineral is tofu or soybeans, spinach, salmon, and nuts.

Vitamin D

Vitamin D, like calcium, is essential for bone and muscle health. Deficiencies in vitamin D a common and lead to poor muscle health in otherwise healthy people. If you have sarcopenia, it is important you are getting enough vitamin D through your diet or supplementation.

Good sources of vitamin D are mushrooms, fatty fish, cheese, and fortified milk.

HMB

HMB is short for beta-hydroxy beta-methyl butyrate, an acid that naturally occurs in your body when leucine is broken down. HMB supplementation allows you to take in more protein than you would be able to by eating whole foods. One gram of HMB taken three times a day is equal to about 600 grams of protein.

HMB is not approved or regulated by the FDA and you should not take this before talking with your doctor.

Zinc

Zinc is an immune-boosting, vital mineral that helps muscles grow when used in conjunction with exercise. It is needed for your body to make and use protein. A deficiency of zinc could lead to impaired immune function, loss of appetite, and poor wound healing. Rich sources of zinc include red meat, legumes, chia seeds, and whole grains.

Talk To Your Doctor

Before adding any new supplements to your diet, always talk to your doctor or registered dietitian about sarcopenia treatment. These vitamins, minerals, and supplements could help you manage or even pre-vent the symptoms of sarcopenia. It's not too late to start an exercise program and take charge of your nutrition.

CHAPTER FOUR

Aging and Why Do We Age?

Aging can be defined as a "time-dependent functional decline that affects most living organisms". Aging has many causes and already in 1990 Medvedev had identified 300 theories of aging. The following "hallmarks" of aging have been proposed:

1. Deregulated nutrient sensing;

2. Loss of proteostasis (protein homeostasis);

3. Mitochondrial dysfunction;

4. Stem cell exhaustion;

5. Altered intracellular communication;

6. Telomere attrition;

7. Cellular senescence;

8. Genomic instability and

9. Epigenetic alterations.

In summary, many mechanisms or hallmarks contribute to aging and the causes and time courses of aging differ from organ to organ and in-between species.

Global Aging Trends and How Do They Affect Societies?

The world's population is aging on average because fewer babies are born and because people live longer. As a consequence, the fraction of older people increases worldwide. In 2015, over 20% of the populations in Japan, Germany, and Italy were aged 65 years and older. At the same time, people aged 15-64 years have decreased so that fewer working young must now support more individuals aged 65 years and older. This demographic shift is a major challenge for all societies affected by it.

Effects of Aging

Aging affects all body organs and systems is the skeletal muscle. As we age our muscles undergo progressive changes, primarily involving loss of muscle mass and strength. The age-related loss of muscle function is known as Sarcopenia, derived from the Greek words for flesh (sarcos) and loss (penia) and its definition includes loss of muscle strength and power, as well as reduced function. It occurs with increasing age and is a major component in the development of frailty.

The loss of muscle mass during the aging process is important clinically as it reduces strength and exercise capacity, both of which are needed to perform activities of daily living.

Can we slow the effects of aging?

Though aging is inevitable, it's possible to slow down some of the effects. You can do this by following healthy lifestyle habits.

Here's how to slow aging:

- Eat a nutritious diet. Focus on fruits, vegetables, whole grains, and lean protein. Limit processed foods.

- Stay active. Exercise reduces the physical and mental effects of aging. Aim for 30 minutes a day, 5 days a week.

- Avoid tobacco. Tobacco speeds up aging. Quitting is often difficult, but a doctor can help create a cessation plan that works for you.

- Drink alcohol in moderation. Alcohol increases your risk of chronic disease.

- Attend regular checkups. Routine checkups with a doctor are the best way to prevent or treat disease early.

- Know your family history. Discuss your family's health history with your doctor to have appropriate screening or get early treatment for potential chronic diseases.

- Engage your brain. Protect your cognitive function by doing brain exercises.

- Wear sunscreen. Sunscreen protects your skin from UV radiation, which can lead to premature aging.

Aging is likely caused by a combination of reasons. Some theories suggest cells have a predetermined lifespan, while others claim it's caused by error and damage. Other theories say that aging is due to genetic, evolution, or biochemical reactions.

Aging is normal, but following a healthy lifestyle may help you live longer. Habits like eating well, exercising regularly, and wearing sunscreen can reduce your risk of disease and improve your quality of life.

CHAPTER FIVE

Sarcopenia – consequences

Sarcopenia is not a disease but rather refers specifically to the universal, involuntary decline in lean body mass that occurs with age, primarily due to the loss of skeletal muscle. Systematic review and meta-analyses among Japanese community-dwelling older adults suggest the prevalence of sarcopenia (9.9% overall: 9.8% among men, and 10.1% among women), providing valuable information in addressing sarcopenia prevention in the older community. A narrative review published in the International Journal of Molecular Sciences (2020) provides new evidence regarding the mechanisms, evaluation and detection methods, and spinal sarcopenia treatment modalities.

Losing muscle mass and becoming weaker during aging have consequences for health. They are:

    1. Frailty – Sarcopenia is associated with frailty which overlaps with sarcopenia but additionally includes weight loss, exhaustion, slow walking speed, and low physical activity.

2. Mortality – Low strength at middle and older ages is associated with increased all-cause and cancer mortality.

3. Daily living tasks – Lower grip strength during middle age is associated with more problems of solving daily life tasks 25 years later, suggesting that sarcopenia increases the risk of not being able to live an independent life.

4. Falls – Especially leg weakness is associated with an increased risk of falls.

Frailty, high mortality, the inability to carry out daily living tasks, and the risk of falling are some of the health issues associated with sarcopenia.

The loss of lean body mass reduces function, and the loss of approximately 40% of lean body mass is fatal. It has been attributed to a reduction of muscle size as well as a reduction in satellite cells (a stem cell that lies adjacent to skeletal muscle fiber and plays a role in muscle growth, repair, and regeneration), mitochondrial numbers, and elasticity.

Sarcopenia is seen in increasing numbers with advancing age but is not universal.

Sarcopenia varies in degree of physical activity, gender, and race.

Sarcopenia has a marked effect on function in all activities of daily living, contributing (along with the reduction in balance) to reduced gait speed, falls, and fractures. The combination of osteoporosis and sarcopenia results in the frailty which frequently occurs in the elderly population.

A systematic review and meta-analysis suggest a higher prevalence of Sarcopenia in individuals with Cardiovascular disease (CVD), dementia, diabetes mellitus, and respiratory disease.

Age-related Changes in Muscle Structure

With increasing age, we lose muscle mass: lean muscle mass contributes up to 50% of total body weight in young adults, but this decreases to 25% by 75 to 80 years[10]. Typical muscle changes with age:

Reduced muscle mass (replaced by increased fat mass)

Reduction in lower limb muscle cross-sectional area has been observed to begin in early adulthood and accelerate beyond 50 years of age. This reduction in muscle cross-sectional area is associated with decreases in contractile structures accompanied by increases in non-contractile structures such as fat and connective tissue. A cross-sectional study suggested that the older inpatient showed an increase in the intramuscular quadricep muscle adipose tissue approx 1.7 times that of the healthy older individuals. Also, the study observed increased intramuscular adipose tissue with older inpatients who were unable to walk independently as compared to older inpatients who were able to walk freely.

Reduced muscle strength

The total number of muscle fibers is significantly reduced with age, beginning at about 25 years and progressing at an accelerated rate thereafter The decline in muscle cross-sectional area is most likely due to decreases in total fiber number, especially type II fast-twitch glycolytic fibers. This results in reduced muscle power. A study examining 1-year changes in the physical functioning of older people using the ICF framework showed a significant decrease in muscle strength (both hip abductors and knee extensors) walking capacity, speed, mobility, sit-to-stand performance, upper extremity function, and balance performance at the end of 1 year.

1. Changes in Muscle Fiber Size

Elderly individuals often fall because of poor muscle strength and reduced balancing ability related to muscle aging. Types IIA and IIB muscle fibers decrease with age in the area percentage, fiber number percentage, and mean fiber area, whereas Type I fibers increase in area and number but not in size. Morphologically, Type II fibers appeared smaller and flatter. Investigations suggest deterioration in muscle quality and balancing coordination in elderly patients. A research done provided data to help determine treatments for reversing muscle fiber changes and reducing the number of falls and related fractures in patients. The reduction in the number of muscle fibers contributes more to the decrease of whole muscle cross-sectional area than does the reduction in the area of individual fibers. The individual fast-twitch type II fibers decrease in the cross-sectional area suggest that the relative contribution of fast-twitch type II fibers to force generation is less in the older adult.

2. Motor Unit Number and Size

In the aged motor unit there is decreased in the number of functional motor units associated with the enlargement of the cross-sectional area of the remaining units. This motor unit remodeling is achieved by selective denervation of muscle fibers, (especially type 2 b fibers) followed by re innervation by axonal spouting from juxtaposed innervation units.

The majority of the literature indicates that muscle fiber loss is due to a loss in motor neurons. There is consistent denervation and reinnervation of the muscle fiber throughout one's lifespan, but in the aged, denervation appears to outpace reinvention.

Data indicate that a 60-year-old has approximately 25-50% fewer motor neurons than a 20-year-old, with the greatest losses in distal fast-twitch motor neurons.

With the loss of the motor neuron, the denervated fast-twitch muscle fibers that were attached to it are either permanently denervated and undergo apoptosis, or are reinvented with a different motor neuron most likely that of a slow-twitch neuron, potentially making the fiber take on slow-twitch characteristics.

Effects of Endocrine Changes on Muscle

With increased age, the following changes in endocrine function result in sarcopenia:

- Increased insulin resistance
- Decreased growth hormone
- Reduction in estrogen and testosterone
- Vitamin D deficiency
- Increased parathyroid hormone
- Conditions Associated with Impairment of Skeletal Function
- Diabetes
- Metabolic syndrome
- Chronic Obstructive Airways Disease (COPD)
- Congestive Cardiac Failure
- Osteoarthritis
- Parkinsons
- Cancer
- Stroke
- Chronic Kidney Disease

Gender differences

Increased muscle quality from resistance training is a common finding in older adults, and in men, there appears to be no difference in young versus old, but there is a study that suggests that older women have a blunted response relative to younger women.

Frequency of resistance training

Studies have demonstrated that resistance training regimes performed once, twice, or even three times a week all result in strength improvements.

Length of the training program

Many studies clearly demonstrate that older people who participate in resistance training programs lasting at least 6 to 12 weeks will show an increase in both strength and mobility function.

Dietary Advice

The Society for Sarcopenia, Cachexia, and Wasting convened an expert panel to develop nutritional recommendations for sarcopenia prevention and management. This panel concluded that for preventing and treating this condition key components are

- protein and energy intake
- both resistance and aerobic exercise

The greatest effects are observed when resistance training and high protein diets are combined and appear to act synergistically.

- Specifically, consuming 20-35 grams of protein per meal is advised, as such amounts provide sufficient amino acid content to maximize MPS, thus minimizing age-related muscle loss. eg

- Chicken Breast: 23.1 g, Protein Per 100 g.

- Canned Tuna: 23.6 g, Protein: Per 100 g.

- Cocoa: 20 g, Protein: Per 100 g.

- Cheddar Cheese: 24.9 g, Protein Per 100 g.

- Beef Jerky: 33.2 g. Protein Per 100 g.

- Additionally, patients with sarcopenia are recommended to consume 1.0 – 1.2 g/kg (body weight)/day

Is there a role for supplements?

There is some evidence suggesting that additional supplementation with the amino acid Leucine (or its metabolite HMB) could potentially increase the effects of resistance training to combat sarcopenia. A randomized double-blind study has found that supplementation with l-leucine can be used in the treatment of sarcopenia in older individuals.

Imagine what happens when you can combat the effects of aging and maintain your muscle mass and strength well into your golden years. While resistance training and a balanced diet are crucial components in the fight against sarcopenia, the addition of certain supplements may give you an extra edge in this battle.

Visualize yourself as a wise, seasoned warrior, armed with the knowledge and tools to keep your body strong and resilient. One of these powerful tools is the amino acid Leucine, or its metabolite HMB.

These supplements have shown promising results in enhancing the effects of resistance training, helping you to build and maintain muscle mass even as you age.

In a randomized double-blind study, researchers uncovered that supplementation with l-leucine can be an effective treatment for sarcopenia in older people. This means that by incorporating leucine into your daily routine, alongside your regular exercise regimen, you can take a proactive approach to combat muscle loss and maintain your strength and vitality.

But how does leucine work its magic? This essential amino acid plays a crucial role in stimulating muscle protein synthesis, the process by which your body builds and repairs muscle tissue.

By providing your body with an extra boost of leucine, you can improve this process and keep your muscles strong and healthy.

Think of your muscles as a fortress, with leucine acting as the reinforcements that help to fortify and protect your body's defenses against the effects of aging. With each passing year, your fortress may face challenges, but with the right tools and strategies, you can keep it standing tall and strong.

"The greatest wealth is health." - Virgil

As you begin on your progress to combat sarcopenia, remember that supplements like leucine and HMB are just one piece of the puzzle. A well-rounded approach that includes regular resistance training, a balanced diet rich in protein, and plenty of rest and recovery is essential for optimal results.

Start by incorporating leucine or HMB supplements into your daily routine, following the recommended dosage on the product label. Be sure to choose a high-quality supplement from a reputable manufacturer to ensure purity and potency.

Next, focus on your resistance training program. Aim for at least two to three sessions per week, targeting all major muscle groups.

Use a combination of free weights, machines, and bodyweight exercises to keep your workouts varied and challenging.

Finally, don't forget the importance of rest and recovery. Allow your body adequate time to repair and rebuild between workouts, and prioritize sleep as an essential component of your overall health and well-being.

CHAPTER SIX

Causes of Sarcopenia

Sarcopenia, also known as muscle loss, is a common condition that affects 10% of adults who are over 50 years old. While it can decrease life expectancy and quality of life, there are actions you can take to prevent and even reverse the condition.

Although some of the causes of sarcopenia are a natural consequence of aging, others are preventable. In fact, a healthy diet and regular exercise can reverse sarcopenia, increasing lifespan and quality of life. This chapter explains what causes sarcopenia, and lists many ways you can fight it.

Sarcopenia literally means "lack of flesh." It's a condition of age-associated muscle degeneration that becomes more common in people over the age of 50. After middle age, adults lose 3% of their muscle strength every year, on average. This limits their ability to perform many routine activities.

Unfortunately, sarcopenia also shortens life expectancy in those it affects, compared to individuals with normal muscle strength.

Sarcopenia is caused by an imbalance between signals for muscle cell growth and signals for teardown. Cell growth processes are called "anabolism," and cell teardown processes are called "catabolism". For example, growth hormones act with protein-destroying enzymes to keep muscle steady through a cycle of growth, stress or injury, destruction, and then healing.

This cycle is always occurring, and when things are in balance, muscle keeps its strength over time. However, during aging, the body becomes resistant to the normal growth signals, tipping the balance toward catabolism and muscle loss.

Your body normally keeps signals for growth and teardown in balance. As you age, your body becomes resistant to growth signals, resulting in muscle loss. Although sarcopenia is caused by age, there are factors associated with aging that affect muscle strength and tone.

Muscle decline starts to happen from the age of 40. In the years between 40 and 70, a person can expect to experience about 8% muscle loss every 10 years.

After age 70, muscle deterioration occurs faster, and without intervention, you can lose approximately 15% of muscle mass every decade.

Factors that can affect muscle loss in the elderly include hormonal imbalances, inflammation, increased fat mass, and nutrient deficiencies.

Let's look briefly at some of the main reasons for loss of muscle strength with aging.

Sedentary lifestyle and lack of physical activity

Not being physically active enough is one reason for muscle loss after age 50. Studies have shown that a sedentary lifestyle can result in muscle atrophy in older people. Low physical activity negatively affects skeletal muscle mass and strength. This can cause weakened muscles, especially in the lower limbs.

Disuse of muscle is one of the strongest triggers of sarcopenia, leading to faster muscle loss and increasing weakness. Bed rest or immobilization after an injury or illness leads to rapid loss of muscle. Although less dramatic, two to three weeks of decreased walking and other regular activity is also enough to decrease muscle mass and strength. Periods of decreased activity can become a vicious cycle. Muscle strength decreases, resulting in greater fatigue and making it more difficult to return to normal activity.

In fact, lack of physical activity is seen as one of the main causes of sarcopenia. A sedentary lifestyle can also increase your risk of other chronic diseases such as heart disease, diabetes, and arthritis.

Poor diet lacking nutrients

A diet lacking in amino acids, protein, and other important nutrients can speed up the development of sarcopenia.

Researchers have found that even elderly people who have a healthy body mass index (BMI) may still be lacking in essential nutrients to prevent muscle loss. A diet providing insufficient calories and protein results in weight loss and diminished muscle mass.

Unfortunately, low-calorie and low-protein diets become more common with aging, due to changes in sense of taste, problems with the teeth, gums, and swallowing, or increased difficulty shopping and cooking. To help prevent sarcopenia, scientists recommend consuming 25–30 grams of protein at each meal.

Some researchers have suggested that people over 60 should increase their protein intake to help prevent sarcopenia symptoms. Increasing dietary protein helps to build muscle mass and increase muscle strength.

Later in this book, you will learn about the best foods to build muscle mass after age 60.

Chronic inflammation

One of the reasons why you could lose muscle mass and strength in later years is due to long-term inflammation. After injury or illness, inflammation sends signals to the body to tear down and then rebuild the damaged groups of cells.

Chronic or long-term diseases can also result in inflammation that disrupts the normal balance of teardown and healing, resulting in muscle loss. For example, a study of patients with long-term inflammation resulting from chronic obstructive pulmonary disease (COPD) also showed that patients had decreased muscle mass.

Examples of other diseases that cause long-term inflammation include rheumatoid arthritis, inflammatory bowel diseases like Crohn's disease or ulcerative colitis, lupus, vasculitis, severe burns, and chronic infections like tuberculosis.

A study of 11,249 older adults found that blood levels of C-reactive protein, an indicator of inflammation, strongly predicted sarcopenia, This study found that sarcopenia is one of the results. The aging process can cause an increase in low- grade inflammation. This can affect muscle protein metabolism and result in skeletal muscle wasting and poor strength.

In fact, chronic inflammation can make it difficult to reverse sarcopenia. Scientists have found that inflammation both causes muscle waste and prevents new muscle tissue growth.

Stress

Stress can cause a number of health problems, with age-related muscle waste being just one of them. The reason why stress can be a reason for losing muscle mass is that it affects your hormones. A 2018 review found that chronic stress causes disorders that impact your muscle mass. Anxiety, depression, and obesity can result in stress-related osteosarcopenic obesity, a condition that causes weak bones and low muscle mass.

Sarcopenia is also more common in a number of other health conditions that increase stress on the body. For example, people with chronic liver disease, and up to 20% of people with chronic heart failure, experience sarcopenia.

In chronic kidney disease, stress on the body and decreased activity lead to muscle loss. Cancer and cancer treatments also place great stress on the body, resulting in sarcopenia.

In addition to aging, sarcopenia is accelerated by low physical activity, insufficient calorie, and protein intake, inflammation and stress.

CHAPTER SEVEN

The Biological Mechanism of Sarcopenia.

The biological mechanism of sarcopenia appears to be in the decreased ability of satellite cells to propagate themselves. Satellite cells are required to fuse into skeletal muscle fibers and help in settings where repair and regeneration are required. Therefore, aging muscle loses its ability to respond to anabolic stimuli, such as insulin, growth hormone, and amino acids. Catabolic stimuli may also play a role: the inflammatory IL-6, IL1-Ra, and TNF-alpha are elevated in elderly people with significant sarcopenia. Many anabolic stimuli are withdrawn in the elderly population. Decreased protein intake in the elderly plays a role: 1/3 of men over the age of 60 eat less than the recommended dietary allowance (RDA) of 0.8 g/kg. A decline in exercise, a potent stimulus to protein synthesis, also contributes. Hormonal factors may be involved, such as decreased levels of sex hormones, growth hormones, and decreased insulin.

Depleted muscles atrophy and are replaced by connective tissue, though the mechanism in sarcopenia may be different than that seen in other settings of "muscle atrophy" since in younger individuals there is not an obvious problem with the satellite cells. Type II muscle fibers atrophy more so than type I.

Individuals' dietary needs change with age. Older adults may require less energy, experience less efficient absorption and utilization of many nutrients, and have different nutrient requirements due to chronic conditions and medications. These changes result in older adults needing a nutrient-dense diet. Unfortunately, it can be challenging for this population to obtain such a nutrient-dense diet because it involves overcoming barriers such as loss of appetite, changes in taste and smell, oral health decline, mobility constraints, and lower incomes.

Some dietary changes are recommended based on the available data. Older adults should be encouraged to eat:

- more fruits and vegetables, especially orange and dark green vegetables, to increase intakes of vitamin C, carotenoids, folate, vitamin B6, magnesium, potassium, and dietary fiber;

- more low-fat dairy to improve intakes of magnesium, calcium, potassium, and vitamins B12 and D;

- more whole grains, including more fortified breakfast cereals, to increase intakes of vitamin B6, crystalline vitamin B12, magnesium, and dietary fiber;

- fewer foods high in sugar, solid fats, sodium; and fewer refined grains.

Factors That Contribute To Sarcopenia.

Many factors contribute to sarcopenia. In the following, five key factors will be discussed:

1. **Loss of motor neurons and muscle fibers and muscle fiber atrophy.**

Cross-sectional studies suggest that during normal aging, spinal limb motor neurons, and up to half of the vastus lateral muscle fibers are lost. The problem with these studies is, that the individuals were born up to 70 years apart.

Because of that, the lower motor neuron and muscle fiber numbers might be due to different environmental conditions and not due to a loss of neurons and fibers during aging. In support of the latter, Nilwik et al did not observe substantially fewer muscle fibers in older individuals. However, both Nilwik et al and Lexell et al reported muscle fiber atrophy, especially of type II fibers.

2. Anabolic resistance.

Muscle fibers hypertrophy if protein synthesis exceeds breakdown. In fasted muscle protein turnover does not differ much between young and old muscle. However, when stimulated with essential amino acids, resistance exercise, or insulin, young muscles increase protein synthesis more than old muscles. The reduced response of old muscle to anabolic stimuli has been termed "anabolic resistance". Such anabolic resistance of old muscle, however, is not always observed.

3. Impaired regeneration due to reduced stem cell function.

Skeletal muscle has an enormous capacity to regenerate after injury. Such regeneration is dependent on satellite cells, the resident stem cells of skeletal muscle. When compared to young, old human muscle has fewer satellite cells and regenerates less e.g. after immobilization atrophy. This suggests that satellite cells are a key factor in sarcopenia. However, removing almost all satellite cells from young mouse muscles has hardly any effect on skeletal muscle aging which seems surprising. A possible explanation is that satellite cell-depleted muscles of caged mice can age normally. However, in a real-life scenario, any injury or immobilization atrophy will cause a problem becausemuscles cannot fully regenerate without satellite cells. Thus, satellite cells are probably important for the aging of a normally "used" human skeletal muscle.

4. Low-grade inflammation.

Aging is associated with chronically increased levels of pro-inflammatory cytokines such as interleukin-6 (IL6) and tumor necrosis factor-α(TNF-α). This is described as chronic low-grade inflammation or as a chronic low-grade inflammatory profile (CLIP) In older men and women, higher levels of pro- inflammatory cytokines are associated with sarcopenia and a greater risk of losing muscle mass and strength. Whilst the mechanisms are not fully understood, chronic low-grade inflammation seems to contribute to sarcopenia.

5. Testosterone in hypogonadal men.

The concentrations of the male sex hormone testosterone vary at all ages and decline with aging. Low testosterone affects muscle mass because giving between 25 and 600mg of testosterone enanthate to men with suppressed endogenous testosterone increases the cross-sectional area of muscle fibers in a dose-dependent manner. Thus, low testosterone concentrations contribute to sarcopenia in hypogonadal males.

In summary, muscle size and function vary greatly at all ages and decline with normal aging, which is termed sarcopenia. Sarcopenia is a slow process caused by many factors including a loss of motor neurons and muscle fibers, anabolic resistance, an impaired regeneration, chronic low-grade inflammation, and a decline of testosterone in hypogonadal men.

CHAPTER EIGHT

How Can We Prevent Sarcopenia

What we know is, regardless of beliefs, religions, and ideas, you are born, is you live and you die. I make it sound short and that is because it is. We have a short existence here on Earth that we know of. After which point, the body you inhabit becomes worm food. Because life is so short, it is important that you can function and enjoy it as much as possible. To really enjoy life, you will obviously need to be strong and fit. The idea of being strong and fit will vary in people's individual opinions. Some of us have no care for bulking up and lifting tractor-trailers and some of us can care less about being able to sprint or jump higher than another person. That's just fine. However, we should all agree that being able to move in different directions as fast as you could (or can) while in your "20s". Also, maintaining optimal posture is a good thing no matter what we think strong and fit means. These features are major parts of quality in life. So, if we want to hold on to the quality of life we will need to hold on to our strength. Since we are born to move quickly in multiple directions and if we stop doing so we lose the ability (sometimes forever) we need to fend our bodies from the effects of sarcopenia as long as possible.

Sarcopenia is a term utilized to define the loss of muscle mass and strength that occurs with aging. That's right, while you get older you lose muscle mass and strength, and with that comes the loss of speed, flexibility, and coordination.

The good thing for us is we can slow these effects to a crawl. The bad thing is this is the natural progression of your life after your physical peak. You will hit the age of your individual top performance physically. After this point, the potential begins to slowly (and for coach potato types--quickly) decline.

Usually, a person will unknowingly hit his or her climax of physical fitness and after cycles of ridiculous diets and overhyped fat-burning supplements, he will begin to lose large amounts of potential to get lean, strong, and fit.

A good example of this is competitive athletes such as Misty May and Kerri Walsh. They hit their physical peak and are now going through a decline of physical potential. However, they are becoming wiser in their sport. The same can be said about legends like Michael Jordan. Michael Jordan hit his peak at a young age in the NBA. Later Jordan retired and returned to basketball to find he was not in peak potential condition to outrun and outmaneuver his younger opponents. However, he came back wiser and took advantage of outside shots and young arrogance that thrived in his opponents. A smart coach once told me the phrase "if I only knew then what I know now..." That phrase sums up what most of us feel as we get older and lose fitness potential. The great thing about these examples is they are athletes who have not lost much muscle mass and strength while they age. In this chapter, I will show you how to hold onto muscle mass and strength even if you are not an elite-level athlete.

Sarcopenia brings about fragility later in life. The principle SAID hits hard here. The body needs to be stimulated and overloaded to maintain muscle mass, flexibility, speed, and dexterity. Those who become obese while growing older are in more danger of becoming what we call "fat-frail". Think on the lines of the fat guy on one of those little scooter things puttering around a super Wal-Mart. He looks like a massive heart attack waiting to happen.

When I say frail, I mean the loss of the type IIa muscle fibers. I would add the loss of type IIb muscle fibers is also a pretty bad deal. For those who do not know, the type II muscle fibers are fast-twitch fibers. They are responsible for speed, agility, and maintaining strength. Not only that, it's the type II fibers that allow for a person to not only become lean and solid "tone", but allows that person to hold on to that look (seriously looking good naked). So, to fend off sarcopenia and remain strong and fit you need to hold onto and recruit fast-twitch type II muscle fibers. More specifically, you need to lift heavier weights and do faster-moving short-duration energy system training. Please do not confuse with riding your bike with family on the weekends down a street, or going into one of those dances and lift classes at your gym, which is fully equipped with a bubbly, springy, over-caffeinated instructor.

The declining ability to remodel these important muscle proteins may therefore play a role in the development of muscle wasting, metabolic abnormalities, and impaired physical functioning seen in old age. Simply saying the testosterone levels and GH levels will drop. This isn't good for males or females. It's what makes maintaining muscle easier. It is what allows you to eat like a horse and work out like one. It is also the major factor in sex drive. Now, where the hell is

HOW TO FIGHT MUSCLE LOSS AS YOU AGE?

your quality of life if you have no sex drive? We are really looking at the decline in DHEA (dehydroepiandrosterone-sulfate), testosterone, and insulin- induced IGF-1 (growth factor). To slow this proponent once again, lift and lift heavy. Do short-duration energy system work. Finally, eat like you want to maintain muscle mass and look good naked. For the vegans and vegan wannabes (you know the types that eat salad all day but don't mind an egg, or don't consider fish and chicken meat... ah if stupidity could kill...). You need protein and good animal sources of eating. That's right sacrifice healthy animals to maintain your sex drive. Reduced protein synthesis leads to atrophy in muscle mass and degradation in testosterone production. I'm not going to outline all the needs here.

Sarcopenia has been linked to several chronic afflictions that are common among the aged, including osteoporosis, insulin resistance, and arthritis. To keep the skeletal system healthy the same methods have to be applied as recruiting muscle. You have to lift heavyweights. The bones are just like muscles when it comes to gaining strength. The strength is very specific to the exercises used. So don't expect leg extensions to keep your spine strong, in fact, don't expect a ridiculous exercise like leg extensions to do anything more than cause knee pain. You will need to get moving with multi-joint exercises (i.e. deadlifts, squats, pushups, etc.).

To wrap this up, you will always have type I muscle fibers. These muscle fibers are simply for endurance and are slow-twitch in nature. They are not hard to maintain or recruit. For quality life and body you will need to recruit type II muscle fibers. These guys give you strength, power, and speed. They will keep you from being a frail and slow-moving person who is just hanging on to life. Instead, they will allow you to maintain a great body and enjoy the quality and function of life. Below I listed some quick guidelines to get you on track and fending off sarcopenia. Be smart and follow them.

1. Eat a proper omnivore diet.

2. Move your body in all "planes of motion". You are not a 2D cartoon move 3D.

3. Master the primal movements used in life (squats, pushups, chin-ups, dips, deadlift, lunges, and twist)

4. Lift a weight that is heavy enough to cause a great deal of effort to get the number of reps you planned to do. In other words, don't grab the fluorescent pink dumbbells and start doing ballerina squats.

5. Be smart when doing cardio. Unless you have an interest in doing a marathon event do not waste time training that way. Move fast as possible for short intervals.

No current intervention will bring back significant numbers of muscle fibers or satellite cells lost during aging. However, progressive resistance (strength) training in combination with nutritional interventions can increase the cross- sectional area and function of muscle fibers. Key anti-sarcopenia interventions are:

1. **Progressive resistance (strength) training.**

Resistance training increases muscle protein synthesis, the size especially of type II fibers, muscle size, and strength in old men and women. The increase of muscle protein synthesis after resistance exercise depends on the mechanistic target of rapamycin (mTOR), as blocking mTOR with rapamycin prevents the increase of muscle protein synthesis after resistance exercise. Even over 90- year-old individuals can increase their muscle function through resistance training. This identifies progressive resistance training as an effective intervention to improve muscle strength in old men and women. Suitable resistance training programs must be safe, effective, and attractive for this cohort. However, the muscle size and strength adaptation to resistance training vary greatly in humans. Thus, the same type of resistance training might increase muscle function in some patients but might not have any measurable effect in others. In another study all subjects improved at least one measure of muscle size or function after 12-24 weeks of resistance exercise, suggesting that all subjects benefit from a suitably designed resistance training program.

2. Protein and other nutrients.

The key "anabolic nutrient" is protein, which is digested into amino acids. Essential amino acids, and especially leucine, stimulate muscle protein synthesis through mTOR because the mTOR inhibitor rapamycin can block an amino acid-stimulated increase of human muscle protein synthesis. There is no conclusive evidence for an "anabolic window" during or around a bout of resistance exercise, but ingesting 20-40g of protein before, during, and/or after resistance exercise should stimulate protein synthesis near-maximally. Finally, what protein is best? Proteins with a high leucine content that are easily digested have the highest protein quality as measured by the digestible indispensable amino acid score (DIAAS). Whey and generally dairy proteins have high DIAAS scores and are therefore especially recommended to promote muscle anabolism.

3. Other nutrients and ergogenic aids.

Creatine, vitamin D supplements, ω-3 polyunsaturated fatty acids (PUFA, fish oil), or β-hydroxy-β-methyl butyrate (HMB), a leucine-related metabolite may all further enhance muscle anabolism.

4. Pharmaceutical treatments

In men, testosterone supplementation especially of hypogonadal men is an effective treatment to preserve muscle mass but the side effects and the safety are insufficiently researched. β-agonists as well as myostatin antibodies/inhibitors can successfully be used to increase muscle size and function. These treatments might be used in cases where resistance exercise is impractical or ineffective or where maximal anabolism is needed, for example, to treat hospitalized hip fracture patients.

5. Experimental treatments

Studies have shown that the removal of senescent cells, or a short-term induction of the stem-cell inducing Yamanaka factors, can delay or reverse both organismal and skeletal muscle aging.

Treatment Tips

Protein supplementation, exercise, and vitamin D are the established, basic treatments for sarcopenia, even within the conventional medical system. A closer look:

What to Try First

If you're worried about losing muscle mass and strength as you age, remember that good nutrition, plenty of protein, and a regular strength training program are essential therapies. They'll not only help to prevent sarcopenia, but will help keep you healthier, leaner, and free from chronic disease;

1. Make sure you're getting enough dietary protein. Eat more fish, eggs, poultry, and lean red meat. If tolerated, also include fermented dairy, milk, and legumes. Meal replacement shakes can also be a good way to make sure you're getting enough protein into your diet.

2. Next, focus on strength training. The combination of increased protein and strength training will increase muscle mass and strength more than either therapy alone.

These simple steps will provide the foundation for keeping you strong, mobile, and independent. Extra supplementation with protein powder such as whey protein (25-30 grams twice a day, including after exercise), leucine (2.5-5 grams per day), and vitamin D (to achieve and maintain blood levels of 50 to 80 ng/mL) can be added for even more powerful sarcopenia support.

Ways To Prevent Muscle Degeneration

Muscle degeneration is a natural part of life. There are a number of reasons why this happens: physical inactivity, lack of calories to sustain muscle, and aging. Age-related muscle degeneration (also known as sarcopenia) affects your ability to do everyday tasks like carrying groceries or even playing with your children or grandchildren.

A steady loss of lean muscle mass is a reality of aging, but you can prevent this by eating well and maintaining a healthy lifestyle. Here are five tips to help you stay healthy and strong.

Work Out Regularly

Adults who are physically inactive lose approximately 3–5% of their muscle mass every decade after the age of 30. This accelerates the older you get.

However, one of the strongest antidotes to age-related muscle degeneration is exercise. For instance, resistance training helps build strength and increase muscle growth. Try these four exercises:

- Knee extensions to strengthen your knees and improve balance

- Half squat using a chair or a wall to increase hip strength

- Upright row with light weights to improve mobility in the shoulder and arms

- Water exercises to increase strength and reduce the impact on joints

Maintain a Balanced Diet

It's no secret that diet and exercise keep our bodies running at optimum levels. However, eating nutritious meals can also help retain muscle. To this effect, it's important that you receive an adequate amount of nutrients. Eating plenty of fruits, veggies, and nuts will provide the protein, carbohydrates, healthy fats, and vitamins that are necessary for muscle retention. Snack on some almonds, walnuts, sunflower seeds, and hemp seeds to get your dose of nutrients. Or prepare them in some tasty dishes like this gluten-free almond cake or these homemade granola bars.

Consume More Protein

Protein provides the necessary amino acids for muscle growth and repair, which may help prevent muscle loss. Besides natural protein-rich foods such as tuna and yogurt, you can supplement your diet with protein powder. While animal- based whey protein powder provides an adequate amount of this macronutrient, there are also many high-quality plant-based protein sources including soy and pea protein powders, chlorella powder, and spirulina. Get your protein fill with this protein açaí bowl or this spirulina smoothie.

Stay Hydrated

We know water is essential to life. Maintaining a healthy lifestyle means staying well-hydrated. However, as we get older, our bodies tend to lose more water, which deprives our muscles of electrolytes. As a result, muscle strength decreases. To keep the cells in your muscles working effectively and optimally, be sure to consume the recommended daily intake of water (which includes drinking water and consuming it through foods): 3.7 liters for men and 2.7 liters for women.

Get Enough Sleep

A major factor in muscle degeneration is a lack of sleep. In fact, rest is just as necessary as proper nutrition and exercise to help muscles grow and repair. Proper sleep increases the synthesis of proteins and decreases the rate of muscle degeneration. The National Sleep Foundation recommends that adults get seven to eight hours of sleep each night for optimum health.

By eating a balanced diet, exercising regularly, and getting a sufficient amount of sleep, you can slow the process of age-related muscle degeneration. That way, you can keep doing the things you enjoy, whether that's gardening, spending time with your family, or taking a leisurely stroll in your neighborhood. Your health is worth it.

Management Of Sarcopenia

For the management of sarcopenia, there is a strong recommendation that individuals with sarcopenia should be enrolled in a resistance exercise program. There is a reasonable amount of evidence that resistance exercise will increase both muscle mass and strength. The use of a protein-rich diet (1 to 1.5 g/day) or protein supplementation received a conditional recommendation based on a small amount of evidence and a previous consensus conference. Higher doses of protein (up to 2 g/day) may be appropriate in persons with severe illness or injury or when there is evidence of a pro-inflammatory/catabolic state. β- hydroxy β-methyl butyrate (HMB) has been shown to improve muscle mass and to preserve muscle strength and function in older people with sarcopenia or frailty. Vitamin D supplementation specifically for sarcopenia was found to have insufficient evidence, though there is evidence that persons with low vitamin D levels may improve their strength with vitamin D supplementation. Similarly, while testosterone can increase muscle mass and strength in older individuals and a meta-analysis has confirmed its safety, the lack of evidence in persons with sarcopenia did not lead to its integration into these recommendations. Preliminary data with anamorelin, a growth hormone secretagogue receptor type 1 (ghrelin receptor) agonist that increases muscle mass but not strength and anti-myostatin antibodies were considered insufficient to make recommendations in favor of their use.

How to Tell if You Are Losing Muscle Mass Due to Aging

Knowing what causes muscle loss with age can help to make lifestyle changes to prevent loss of muscle strength. How can you know you are showing signs of losing muscle mass?

Because sarcopenia develops gradually, it can be difficult to spot its early symptoms. A person experiencing loss of muscle mass in old age may start to drop things, have difficulty picking up familiar objects, or falling more.

As sarcopenia progresses, an older adult may become frailer, lose their fitness, walk slower, and become less active. Stooping is also connected with age- related muscle loss.

There are other medical conditions with symptoms similar to sarcopenia. If you notice a change in your physical abilities or that of an elderly person, you should speak with a doctor.

How to Fight Sarcopenia and Muscle Wasting (Evidence-Based) Exercise

One of the best ways to reverse age-related muscle loss is to have a good physical exercise routine.

Before undertaking any of these physical exercise routines for sarcopenia, it is important to consult with your doctor to get your fitness assessed. This will help to prevent needlessly straining or pulling a muscle.

Here are the best types of exercises to build muscle mass after age 60 or 70.

Resistance or Strength Training to Help Reverse Sarcopenia

A program of strength training can reverse muscle loss in the elderly. Many doctors view this type of training as the best exercise for aging muscles.

Many studies also show that resistance training is an effective weapon in fighting sarcopenia.

The journal Sports Health reports that it is possible to build muscle mass after the age of 60. One study showed that men over 60 increased their muscle mass by 5% daily by lifting 80% of their body weight. Other studies have shown that it's even possible for men over 90 years of age to increase muscle strength.

A 2009 review of 121 trials involving over 6,700 persons found that resistance training is an effective way to build muscle mass and strength in older people. Resistance training improved the gait of elderly people and it was easier for them to get up from a chair.

Studies have shown that a program of targeted training to strengthen all the muscle groups can help to reverse sarcopenia. It is also possible to develop resistance training programs for muscle strength using common household items.

Scientists advise that it's necessary for an elderly person to learn proper lifting and exercise techniques to prevent injury.

Brisk Walking to Boost Muscle Mass

Another type of exercise to prevent muscle wasting and loss of strength in your lower body is to walk.

For many elderly people, walking is one of the best forms of exercise because it is low-impact, good for the heart, and builds muscle strength.

A 2015 study on elderly men and women found that regular walking helped to improve muscle function and prevent sarcopenia. Over a 6-month period, researchers found that walking particularly helped older people who were frail and who had low muscle mass.

One study involving men and women over 60 found that faster walking resulted in a lower risk of sarcopenia.

Daily walking will also help manage weight issues in older people. Find out how much you need to walk every day to lose weight.

Aerobic Training Helps Strengthens Muscles and Prevents Sarcopenia

Cardio exercises are great to help you regain muscle strength and tone if you are over 50.

A 2018 review of the benefits of aerobic training for muscle strength found that it increased metabolism. Researchers found that this had a positive effect on building muscle mass and increasing muscle function.

One study found that cycle exercising helped to increase muscle size in people over the age of 70. Over a 12-week period, the cardiovascular condition, bone health, and muscle mass all improved due to aerobic exercises.

A study carried out in 2018 found that aerobic training can help reverse symptoms of muscle atrophy in the elderly over a 6-week period. Subjects exercised 3 times a week for 45 minutes. Researchers noted that regular exercising helped decrease symptoms of depression and increase muscle mass at the same time.

Food and Nutrition to Help Prevent Muscle Deterioration

Apart from regular exercising to help keep your muscles strong as they age, you also need proper nutrition to build muscle tissue.

A 2016 review into ways to treat sarcopenia found that getting proper nutrition was second in place after resistance training. A healthy diet for building muscle after 60 should include 25-30 g of protein per meal and omega-3 fatty acids.

Proper nutrition can be of great benefit to elderly people experiencing muscle loss.

What are the best foods to include in your diet for sarcopenia? Let's look at the benefits of protein, oily fish, and anti-inflammatory foods to reverse muscle atrophy in the elderly.

Protein Helps Build Muscle Mass After 60

Healthy and strong muscles require protein to prevent deterioration of muscle tissue as you get older.

The Journal of Clinical Medical Research reported on the importance of nutrition for sarcopenia. Researchers found that adequate protein for the elderly and exercise were the 2 most important factors to promote muscle growth.

One study found that women in menopause can prevent muscle loss by consuming around 25-30 grams of high-quality protein with every meal daily. Women who consumed more protein had greater muscle mass than those women who consumed less than the recommended daily intake.

Health professionals recommend consuming an animal or plant-based protein sources that contain all the essential amino acids. For example, one essential amino acid you need to build muscle is leucine. Getting enough protein in your diet can help to prevent or slow down muscle loss due to aging.

Eat Oily Fish to Help Prevent Sarcopenia

There are a number of reasons why fish such as salmon, mackerel, and tuna are good for sarcopenia. Fatty fish not only contains a lot of protein but is also a rich source of omega-3 fatty acids.

The Journal of Frailty & Aging found that omega 3 polyunsaturated fatty acids (PUFAs) provide good nutrition for healthy muscles. There is growing evidence that oily fish rich in omega-3 can be a useful tool in reducing symptoms associated with sarcopenia.

Even though consuming salmon can help stop age-related muscle loss, find out why you should avoid farmed salmon to stay healthy.

Anti-Inflammatory Foods

Because chronic inflammation can be a reason for losing muscle mass as you get older, incorporating inflammation-reducing foods in your diet is a good idea.

A 2017 systematic review found that people with sarcopenia tend to have higher levels of C-reactive protein (CRP). This protein is associated with inflammation in the body.

Some studies have shown that having higher than normal levels of CRP can also lead to sarcopenia and also cause a buildup of plaque in the arteries.

You can find out about some of the best anti-inflammatory foods that can help promote good muscle health. Foods such as ginger, garlic, oily fish, and olive oil all help to lower inflammation in your body.

Other Ways to Help Prevent Sarcopenia

- Regular resistance training and getting enough protein in your diet are two of the best ways of avoiding muscle loss as you age.

- However, there are a few other lifestyle choices that can prevent age- related muscle loss.

- Cut back on alcohol to help stop muscle loss with aging.

- A 2017 study on postmenopausal women found that high alcohol intake was associated with a greater risk of muscle loss after menopause.

- Quit smoking to improve muscle health.

- A meta-analysis of 12 studies found that smoking increases your risk of muscle deterioration in later life.

CHAPTER NINE

How to Fight Sarcopenia with Supplements

In some cases, supplements can help to boost your muscle metabolism and help avoid muscle wasting.

Generally, it is best to get protein, fatty acids, vitamins, and nutrients from your diet. However, these are some supplements that are especially good for building muscle mass.

Protein.

The current Estimated Average Requirement for protein for all adults 19 years and older is 0.66 g/kg/day; however, Tucker indicated that a moderately higher protein intake (1.0–1.3 g/kg/day) may be required for older adults to maintain nitrogen balance due to decreased efficiency of protein synthesis and impaired insulin action. The need for increased protein intake is further supported by the Health, Aging, and Body Composition Study, which found that older adults with the highest intake of protein lost less lean body mass than those with lower protein intakes. However, there is some concern that higher protein intake may increase the risk of toxicity or impaired renal function.

Omega-3 Reduces Inflammation and Helps Prevent Sarcopenia.

Taking omega-3 supplements can help to build muscle mass after age 50 because they help reduce inflammation.

Because farmed salmon isn't recommended and not everyone eats oily fish on a regular basis, supplements are a great way to get your omega-3 intake. Among adults 60 years and older, the median intake of α-linolenic acid by women was above the Adequate Intake (AI), whereas the median intake by men was not.

Omega-3 fatty acids are associated with protection against heart disease, diabetes, and cognitive decline. Low intake may be partially due to the limited sources in the diet (e.g., fatty fish, flax seeds, and walnuts).

A 2018 review was published on the effects of omega-3 and sarcopenia. Researchers found that taking omega-3 supplements helped prevent muscle loss and improve muscle function.

Vitamin D Helps Increase Muscle and Bone Strength

Taking vitamin D supplements can help to regain muscle tone in later years because they improve bone and muscle metabolism.

Some studies have shown that people who experience age-related muscle deterioration often have a vitamin D deficiency. Researchers noted that addressing vitamin D deficiency was one way of treating sarcopenia symptoms.

Older adults with poor vitamin D intake and status may be due to low intakes of fortified dairy foods and fatty fish, low sun exposure, reduced dermal synthesis of vitamin D3 and decreased capacity of kidneys to convert 25OHD into 1,25- OH2-D. A study of homebound older adults found that about 65 percent had suboptimal concentrations of 25OHD in their blood (less than 50 nmol/L) and 48 percent had intakes below 400 International Units. In addition to its importance to bone status, vitamin D deficiency has been associated with neurological conditions, diabetes, and other metabolic conditions. Increasingly, more nutritionists are recommending that older adults take a vitamin D supplement.

Other studies have found that vitamin D supplements can help treat muscle loss in postmenopausal women. Taking vitamin D helped women over 50 to develop better muscle mass and muscle strength.

Vitamin E.

Vitamin E is important because of its role as an antioxidant and in immune function. There is some controversy over whether the current Recommended Daily Allowance (RDA), 15 mg of α-tocopherol, is too high, as very few individuals are able to meet this recommendation from diet alone. Vitamin E supplements increase α-tocopherol levels while reducing γ-tocopherol, so supplements may not be the healthiest option for increasing intake. Some literature suggests that other tocopherols (found in nuts, seeds, and plant oils) are also important; however, there are no current nutrient recommendations for other forms of vitamin E.

Vitamin B12.

Although the daily intake of total vitamin B12 does not appear to be low for most older adults, dietary intake data may underestimate the number of people who are vitamin B12 deficient given that atrophic gastritis and loss of stomach acid prevent some older adults from absorbing it. As a result, the Institute of Medicine recommended that older adults get their vitamin B12 in the crystalline form such as from fortified foods or supplements.

The Framingham Offspring Study found that non-supplement users had a higher prevalence of low B12 (less than 250 μmol/L) than those who were taking a supplement containing vitamin B12. Vitamin B12 deficiency can lead to peripheral neuropathy, balance disturbances, cognitive disturbances, physical disability, and increased risk of heart disease from high homocysteine. Tucker stated, "It's critical that more attention be given to this important nutrient as many of these symptoms are nonspecific and not always diagnosed correctly".

Vitamin B6.

Vitamin B6 is important for numerous metabolic reactions and health outcomes. Inadequacy may lead to high homocysteine and impaired immune function and has been associated with impaired cognitive function and depression. Data from the Massachusetts Hispanic Elders Study showed that 30 percent of Hispanics and 28 percent of non-Hispanic whites had plasma pyridoxal 5′-phosphate (the active form of vitamin B6 used as a biomarker for vitamin B6 status) concentrations less than 30 nmol/L (an indicator of inadequate status), and 11 percent of Hispanics and 16 percent of nonwhite Hispanics had concentrations less than 20 nmol/L (clinical cutoff level indicating deficient concentrations). Furthermore, pyridoxal 5′-phosphate was associated with depressive symptomatology in this population-based study of older adults.

Dietary fiber.

Fiber is important for intestinal health and protection against heart disease and metabolic syndrome; however, the median intakes of neither men nor women 60 years and older meet the AI.

Excessive intakes.

Excessive intake of some nutrients is also a concern among older adults as it is for the general population.

Sodium.

The Tolerable Upper Intake Level for sodium is 2.3 g/day; however, the 2015 Dietary Guidelines Advisory Committee recommended it should be lowered to 1.5 g/day to reduce the risk of hypertension and heart disease. Men and women over the age of 70 years are exceeding both recommendations; the usual daily mean intake for men and women is 3.0 and 2.4 g, respectively.

Saturated fat.

The Dietary Guidelines for American's recommendation for saturated fat intake is less than 10 percent of energy intake, intending to reduce that recommendation to 7 percent. However, most adults have intakes greater than 10 percent of their energy intake.

Folic acid.

Whereas some adults do not meet the recommended intake levels of folic acid (400 μg), research shows that others are at risk of exceeding the upper level of 1,000 μg per day due to intake of fortified flour and breakfast cereals, and supplement use. More research is needed but high folic acid may contribute to the progression of neurological diseases associated with vitamin B12 deficiency and lead to increased risk of some cancers.

Food intakes.

In order to determine why older adults' nutrient intakes are inadequate, one must review their food intake patterns. The 2011 IOM report Child and Adult Care Food Programs: Aligning Dietary Guidance for All presented the mean daily food group intakes by adults ages 60 years and older as compared to the 2,000-calorie MyPyramid food group pattern. It showed that older adults are not meeting any of the MyPyramid food group recommendations and are exceeding the recommendations for daily intake of solid fats and added sugar.

Why Supplements for Building Muscle Mass and Strength

One way that you can help reverse muscle loss in old age is to take whey protein supplements.

A 2017 randomized controlled trial found that supplementing an elderly person's diet with whey can help to treat symptoms of sarcopenia. Men over the age of 70 took a protein-based supplement for 6 weeks. The results were that the protein supplements helped build muscle mass without exercising. However, when combined with exercising, there was an even greater increase in muscle mass.

Nutritional supplementation is effective in the treatment of sarcopenia in old age, and its positive effects increase when associated with physical exercise. The main limitation of this treatment is the lack of long-term adherence. A healthy diet associated with a physically active lifestyle and possibly with aerobic exercise are the basis of healthy aging, which is the aim of all doctors treating aged people must seek.

CHAPTER TEN

Sarcopenia Treatment

While everyone loses some muscle mass with age, natural sarcopenia treatment can slow or even reverse that loss.

For the elderly, maintaining muscle mass and function is vital to having functional independence. Muscle deterioration can be prevented, decreased, and reversed with the following sarcopenia treatment methods.

1. Exercise Regularly

The adoption of a more sedentary lifestyle is the worst choice to make when it comes to warding off sarcopenia.

When it comes to sarcopenia, exercise has been shown to increase strength, aerobic capacity, and muscle protein synthesis. Exercise also increases muscle mitochondrial enzyme activity in both young and older people.

Resistance exercise, in particular, has been shown to decrease frailty and improve muscle strength in very elderly adults. Exercise is recommended on most days of the week, but a minimum of three times per week is recommended. Slowing muscle loss and prevent sarcopenia is one of the biggest benefits of exercise as we age.

2. Increase Dietary Protein

Protein is the best food for repairing and building muscle fibers. Studies show 12% of men and 24% of women over age 70 eat significantly less optimal protein levels. The recommended protein for healthy adults is 1.2 grams per kilogram of body weight each day. For those with sarcopenia, protein needs are even higher at 1.2 to 1.5 g/kg a day.

3. Choose Protein Wisely

When it comes to positively impacting sarcopenia, what type of protein you consume is crucial. The type of protein you eat also seems to play a role in preventing muscle loss.

Dietary protein is made up of many types of amino acids. The body can make some amino acids on its own, but the rest it must obtain from protein-rich foods. Of the 20 total amino acids, certain ones are considered "essential" because we aren't capable of making them ourselves. Others are "nonessential" because the body can create them by synthesizing other amino acids.

The amino acid leucine has been shown to preserve body muscle. Leucine is an essential amino acid, which means our bodies cannot produce it, so we must get it from dietary sources. A 2010 study showed that the ingestion of leucine- enriched essential amino acids stimulates muscle protein synthesis.

Leucine is found in higher amounts in eggs and products made with milk. It's also found in soybeans and, to a lesser extent, other beans, nuts, and seeds. Therefore, increase protein in your diet with lentils, black beans, or other beans. Also recommended are natto, free-range eggs, and raw goat milk and cheese.

Eating enough protein is necessary to build and maintain healthy muscle mass, while also supporting tendons, ligaments, and other body tissue. Eating protein before and after exercise helps increase muscle recovery and serves as an effective muscle ache treatment.

4. Get More Omega-3s

Omega-3 fatty acids have been found to influence muscle protein metabolism and in the context of human aging. A study found that dietary omega-3 fatty acid supplementation increases the rate of muscle protein synthesis in older adults.

You can consider supplementing your omega-3 acid intake with flaxseed oil.

5. Hormone Balance

Hormonal factors can significantly affect muscle mass. If you're 40 years of age or older, you can have annual blood work done to track your hormone levels.

For women, in particular, hormonal balance can have a direct effect on sarcopenia. Menopause is linked to reduced concentrations of a hormone called estradiol in middle-aged and older women. It's believed that hormonal changes and balance may play a role in sarcopenia in older women.

6. Vitamin D

Studies have shown low blood levels of vitamin D are associated with lower muscle strength and increased body instability in older subjects. (9) Vitamin D deficiency is the most common nutritional deficiency for older adults regardless. Up to 90 percent of adults in the U.S. are believed to have a vitamin D deficiency.

Low vitamin D levels have been associated with sarcopenia. Supplementation of vitamin D in individuals with low levels can help improve muscle function and muscle mass.

7. Eat More Anti-Inflammatory Foods

Chronic inflammation has received attention as a potential contributor to sarcopenia. Eating a more anti-inflammatory diet is crucial. Avoid overly processed, unbalanced foods.

For the sake of improving sarcopenia as well as your overall health, you should increase your intake of anti-inflammatory foods. Green leafy vegetables, blueberries, pineapple, and walnuts are all recommended.

8. Cut Pro-Inflammatory Foods

While eating anti-inflammatory foods, you will also help yourself by foregoing pro-inflammatory foods and substances. Two pro-inflammatory substances are high fructose corn syrup and trans fats. Found in processed foods, these ingredients cause inflammation that contributes to sarcopenia.

Processed foods are also likely to be higher in omega-6 fatty acids, which are necessary but not in large quantities. In excess and without the balance of omega-3s, omega-6 fats actually create inflammation in the body. The typical American diet tends to contain 14–25 times more omega-6 fatty acids than omega-3 fatty acids.

Simple, refined sugars and carbohydrates are more inflammation-causing culprits. Limiting refined grains is another important component of an anti- inflammatory diet.

9. Decrease Alcohol Intake

Drinking too much alcohol over time can weaken the muscles, which is a good reason for all adults to consider their alcohol consumption. If you know you already have sarcopenia, then you want to consider your alcohol consumption even more seriously.

Alcohol abuse appears to affect skeletal muscle severely, promoting its damage and wasting. Alcohol misusers also frequently suffer from low muscle mass and strength, muscle pain, and falls.

Most alcoholic beverages remove critical nutrients from your body. Alcohol, especially in excess, can also contribute to inflammation. With sarcopenia, you want to increase your nutrient intake significantly and decrease bodily inflammation.

10. Stop Smoking

For smokers, here is another great reason to quit. Cigarette smoking is associated with poor lifestyle habits, such as low levels of physical activity and impaired nutrition. In addition, smoking itself is another lifestyle habit that has been found to be associated with sarcopenia.

Studies have found that men and women who were smokers were more likely to have sarcopenia. Electronic cigarettes are also a risk factor for sarcopenia.

CHAPTER ELEVEN

How to Fight Sarcopenia with Exercise

Exercise remains the intervention of choice for sarcopenia, but the translation of research findings into clinical practice is challenging. The type, duration, and intensity of exercise are variable between studies, preventing a standardized exercise prescription for sarcopenia. Lack of exercise is a significant risk factor for sarcopenia and exercise can dramatically slow the rate of muscle loss. Exercise can be an effective intervention because aging skeletal muscle retains the ability to synthesize proteins in response to short-term resistance exercise. Progressive resistance training in older adults can improve physical performance (gait speed) and muscular strength.

Exercise can help prevent sarcopenia.

Several strategies have been evaluated for preventing sarcopenia and its adverse health outcomes, including exercise training, nutritional supplementation, and hormonal therapies. Currently, only physical exercise has shown a positive effect.

Both resistance and aerobic training have been shown to improve overall health and wellness, no matter your age. But the only proven method for the prevention and improvement of sarcopenia is progressive resistance training. A review of 121 sarcopenia research trials concluded that progressive resistance training improves not only muscle strength but also physical performance measures such as gait speed and the ability to rise from a chair. These two performance measures two critical components for fall prevention in older adults.

With progressive resistance training, you need to exercise your muscles against an increasing external force two to three times a week for at least eight to 12 weeks. The program is progressive, meaning that the number of repetitions, sets, or loads should increase gradually over time based on your capabilities and progress.

Types of Sarcopenia Exercises

Progressive resistance training exercises focus on large muscle groups throughout your whole body. Programs vary depending on your individual condition and capabilities, but progressive resistance training may include:

- Push-ups on a counter
- Seated chair push-ups
- Squats with chair touch
- Step-ups
- Standing shoulder rows with anchored resistance

A physical therapist can help you begin a strengthening program customized just for you. If you feel like you're losing strength or muscle mass — whether it's from sarcopenia or any other injury or health issue — schedule an appointment with a physical therapist to improve your movement and ability.

Effect Of Exercise On Sarcopenia

Exercise is essential for health because it increases muscle mass, reduces body fat, and improves muscle strength, endurance, immune function, and the cardiovascular system. Accordingly, exercise should be considered an essential feature of therapeutic strategies targeting age-related sarcopenia. In this chapter, we briefly describe the effects of aerobic, resistance, and combined exercises on age-related sarcopenia.

Aerobic exercise and sarcopenia

Aerobic exercise causes ATP production in mitochondria within skeletal muscle and improves aerobic capacity, metabolic regulation, and cardiovascular function. Furthermore, it contributes to the inductions of mitochondrial biogenesis and dynamics, to the restoration of mitochondrial metabolism, reduces the expressions of catabolic genes, and increases muscle protein synthesis. Previous studies have shown endurance exercise training may suppress the apoptotic pathway in skeletal muscle and that aerobic exercise helps maintain the expression of autophagy protein and may even increase the expressions of autophagy-related proteins in skeletal muscle. In addition, several authors have shown aerobic exercise controls mRNA expression of myostatin. Given that these molecular factors are associated with age-related sarcopenia, it seems aerobic exercise has a protective effect. Indeed, that cycling exercise increased muscle size and strength in both 20-years-old and 74-years- old subjects. Moreover, the 12 weeks of aerobic exercise training enhanced mitochondrial biogenesis and mitochondrial fission protein of older subjects. Collectively, aerobic exercise appears to ameliorate mitochondria-related problems and improve muscle hypertrophy and strength.

Resistance exercise and sarcopenia

Resistance exercise is considered an important strategy for preventing muscle wasting because it stimulates muscle hypertrophy and increases muscle strength by shifting the balance between muscle protein synthesis and degradation towards synthesis. It is known regular resistance exercise increases the sizes and cross-sectional areas of muscle fibers, especially fast-twitch fibers (types IIa and IIx) rather than slow-twitch fibers (type I). Increases in muscle protein synthesis and muscle fibers hypertrophy increase force-generating ability, muscle quality, and physical performance. However, resistance exercise has several limitations. In particular, it has a little effect on the expressions of mitochondrial proteins or their functions, and these are considered potential causes of age-related sarcopenia. Nonetheless, resistance exercise is a meaningful exercise prescription for sarcopenia in terms of improving muscle mass and function. It was shown that progressive resistance training resulted in increased physical performance and peak oxygen uptake. Also reported that 10 weeks of resistance exercise enhanced physical activities, including arm curling and 30-sec chair-stand. In addition, 3 months of resistance exercise improved maximal force production of knee extension and total body fat-free mass. sarcopenia.

Combined exercise and sarcopenia

The majority of studies on the effects of exercise have focused on either aerobic or resistance exercise. As mentioned above, aerobic exercise has little effect on muscle strength or mass compared with resistance exercise, whereas resistance exercise can increase the risk of injury, reduce participation rates, and induce boredom because of the extent of repetition. Also, resistance exercise can be less effective in older individuals because of deficient mTOR signaling, which is involved in muscle protein synthesis. Accordingly, no single type of exercise would seem to address adequately the requirements of therapeutic exercise in age-related sarcopenia, and thus, it has been recommended well-rounded exercise programs consisting of aerobic and resistance exercises should be preferred. For example, a circuit exercise program has been developed that combines these two exercise types. Recently, it was reported that 12 weeks of circuit program improved walking and balancing abilities and isokinetic muscle functions. Also 'multimodal training interventions' conducted on 117 elderly subjects for 6 months improved endurance performance as determined by a 6- min walking test. Collectively, these reports indicate regular combined exercise can be utilized to combat age-related sarcopenia. Further research is needed to determine whether combined exercise retards potential molecular mechanisms of age-related sarcopenia.

Mitochondrial oxidative stress, apoptosis, and dynamics, and mitophagy, myostatin, and inflammatory cytokines are all believed to be associated with age-related sarcopenia. Nevertheless, aerobic, resistance and combined exercise training regimes have been shown to produce the most beneficial preventive and therapeutic effects. Further research is required to elucidate the cellular and molecular mechanisms responsible for the protective effect of regular exercise training on age-induced sarcopenia of skeletal muscles.

Exercise Can Reverse Sarcopenia

The strongest way to fight sarcopenia is to keep your muscles active. Combinations of aerobic exercise, resistance training, and balance training can prevent and even reverse muscle loss. At least two to four exercise sessions weekly may be required to achieve these benefits. All types of exercise are beneficial, but some more than others.

1. Resistance training

Includes weightlifting, pulling against resistance bands, or moving part of the body against gravity.

When you perform resistance exercise, the tension on your muscle fibers results in growth signals that lead to increased strength. Resistance exercise also increases the actions of growth-promoting hormones.

These signals combines to cause muscle cells to grow and repair themselves, both by making new proteins and by turning on special muscle stem cells called "satellite cells," which reinforce existing muscle.

Thanks to this process, resistance exercise is the most direct way to increase muscle mass and prevent its loss.

A study of 57 adults aged 65–94 showed that performing resistance exercises three times per week increased muscle strength over 12 weeks.

In this study, exercises included leg presses and extending the knees against resistance on a weight machine.

2. Fitness Training

Sustained exercise that raises your heart rate, including aerobic exercise and endurance training, can also control sarcopenia.

Most studies of aerobic exercise for the treatment or prevention of sarcopenia have also included resistance and flexibility training as part of a combination exercise program.

These combinations have been consistently shown to prevent and reverse sarcopenia, although it is often unclear whether aerobic exercise without resistance training would be as beneficial.

One study examined the effects of aerobic exercise without resistance training in 439 women over 50 years of age.

The study found that five days per week of cycling, jogging, or hiking increased muscle mass. Women started with 15 minutes of these activities per day, increasing to 45 minutes over 12 months.

3. Walking

Walking can also prevent and even reverse sarcopenia, and it's an activity most people can do for free, anywhere they live.

A study of 227 Japanese adults over 65 years old found that six months of walking increased muscle mass, particularly in those who had low muscle mass. The distance each participant walked was different, but they were encouraged to increase their total daily distance by 10% each month.

Another study of 879 adults over age 60 found that faster walkers were less likely to have sarcopenia.

Exercise is the most effective way to reverse sarcopenia. Resistance training is best to increase muscle mass and strength. However, combination exercise programs, and walking also fight sarcopenia.

Easy Exercises That Fight Muscle Loss as You Age

Sarcopenia, or age-related muscle loss, is a common problem and can be a major cause of pain and discomfort when not managed. Losing muscle mass as we age might seem inevitable, but the truth is, there's a lot that you can do to combat the frustrating condition — and even the smallest bit of effort can make a world of difference.

When it comes to the health of your muscles, bones, and joints, different factors come into play. For one, there's your diet. As you age, it's extremely important to consume adequate protein, omega-3 fatty acids, and vitamin D from healthy, whole-food sources. But on top of diet, the way you exercise is a key ingredient to sustaining healthy, sturdy muscles as time goes along.

Sarcopenia is accelerated by muscle atrophy and lack of use as well as inflammation and stress, so incorporating some exercise into your daily routine will be necessary if you want to stay strong. The good news is, you don't have to overdo it sweating at the gym. The exercises below have all shown to improve muscle mass and even reverse sarcopenia — and they can all be done for free!

Walking

You may think that you're not getting a good workout just by walking because you're not breaking a sweat, but actually, regular walking is really good for your muscles and bones over time. In fact, one study of 227 elderly Japanese adults found that increasing their walking just 10 percent helped to increase muscle mass, specifically in those who previously suffered from low muscle mass.

And don't be afraid to pick up the pace! Another study of adults over 60 found that those who walked faster were less likely to suffer from sarcopenia.

Resistance Exercises

It sounds fancy, but resistance training doesn't require more than your own body weight. Using resistance to engage the muscles causes a surge in growth-promoting hormones that signal the body to produce more muscle tissue. And not only do these signals encourage the growth of new muscle tissue, but they also help to reinforce existing muscle tissue by making it stronger.

One study of adults over the age of 65 showed that resistance training resulted in increased muscle mass after 12 weeks in subjects with limited mobility.

What's more, these individuals also experienced greater flexibility and mobility in their bodies at the end of the study!

Some body-weight resistance exercises you can try include push-ups (try an easier version with your knees on the ground, if you need to!), planks, squats, and lunges. You can find great body-weight resistance workouts on YouTube. And if you're looking to up the ante, you can even try including resistance bands and weights into your routine!

Endurance Exercises

Endurance training refers to aerobic exercise and other sustained movements that raise the heart rate, like biking or swimming, for example. Endurance training is well known for being beneficial to heart health, so it's definitely important to do as you get older.

Promising studies on endurance training for sarcopenia usually combine it with some sort of resistance training. However, one study of women over age 50 found that endurance exercises, namely jogging, cycling, and hiking, increased muscle mass. And what's more, these women were encouraged to start off by adding 15 minutes of exercise, steadily increasing to 45 minutes. That's no time at all!

There you have it. In as little as an extra 15 minutes a day, you can prevent and even reverse the signs of age-related muscle loss at no extra cost to you. All of these exercises can be done for free, so why not start now?

Tips To Fight Sarcopenia Through Proper Exercise And Nutrition

Sarcopenia is a medical condition that comes naturally as we age, but that doesn't mean that we should let it ruin our quality of life. These tips to fight sarcopenia can help.

As time goes by, you notice that your body starts behaving differently. Aging is a natural process, and unfortunately, the associated acute and chronic conditions that come along with it are normal as well. One of the common signs of aging and a common condition that develops in the latter stages of life is called sarcopenia. Simply put, sarcopenia is the loss of muscle mass and bone density, which starts happening after the age of fifty for most people.

Even though sarcopenia is the price we pay for inactivity and a sedentary lifestyle, that doesn't mean that there's nothing you can do to fight its effects. In fact, if you start now, you can build a healthier, stronger body than ever before that will ensure you stay vibrant and healthy throughout your silver years. With that in mind, here are the five tips to fight sarcopenia through proper nutrition and exercise.

Getting slowly back into training

The best way to fight sarcopenia and to stop muscle and bone degradation are to start exercising. However, you can't just spring into action from an otherwise sedentary lifestyle, because you could injure yourself and burn out way before you get the chance to develop long-term habits. Because remember, fitness is a journey, one that begins with you learning to walk before you can run.

So, be sure to start slowly and plan your training journey. You can start by visiting your doctor and having them prescribe you an at-home workout routine. This routine should be light and enjoyable to get your body accustomed to exercise and motivate you to push further. Once you have developed a healthy exercise habit, you can start working on your nutrition.

Developing healthier eating habits

Sarcopenia doesn't have a single point of origin, nor is it something you can overcome just by exercising several times a week. If you are to elevate your overall health, banish unwanted fat, and build functional muscle mass, then you need to start eating well. This process begins with you eliminating all unhealthy foods from your diet and banishing it from your home.

Junk food has no place in your new lifestyle, and you should fill up your pantry and fridge with healthy, wholesome foods from a variety of sources. These should include various vegetables, nuts and seeds, dairy products, lean meats, fish, legumes, and more. That said your key focus should be to get more protein into your diet.

Focusing on protein intake

Protein is so important for fighting sarcopenia that it deserves a separate mention. Most people, young or old, do not get enough protein in their diets on a daily basis. This leads to the overconsumption of other nutrients like carbs and fats, which are not conducive to building lean muscle mass. Remember, protein is the building block of muscle, and you need a protein-focused diet to help build a healthier, stronger body.

That said, getting enough protein on daily basis is difficult. This is why complementing your nutrition with a protein supplement is a good way to get enough protein every day without overconsuming calories. As a senior, you also need to keep in mind that supplementing with protein will alleviate some of the pressure off your digestive system, which can come under stress if you consume too much protein from food.

Progressive overload is the key

Once you have developed the habit of exercising at home and eating properly, you can start upping your training sessions. To build muscle efficiently and effectively, you need to make your workouts progressively more challenging over time. This doesn't mean that you should push yourself beyond your limits, rather, it simply means that incremental progress builds muscle and helps you fuel your fitness goals.

With that in mind, be sure to start adding repetitions to your workouts, prolong your cardio sessions, or even join a local gym. The gym is a controlled environment where you can work out alone or even with a personal trainer who will monitor your progress, keep you safe, and instruct you on the best ways to make your workouts more intense to get the best results.

Making sure your body is recovering

Last but not least, you shouldn't push yourself so hard that your body is unable to recover from the workout. Always keep in mind that muscle growth occurs during the recovery process, not while you're working out. If you want to maximize your performance and achieve your goal, which is to banish sarcopenia, then you need to make sure you're resting properly.

Firstly, know when it's time to stop your workout. Next, make sure you're are sleeping enough so that your body can recuperate. Adhere to proper warm-ups and cool-downs in the gym to stretch your muscles and keep your joints and ligaments flexible and mobile.

Sarcopenia is a medical condition that comes naturally as we age, but that doesn't mean that we should let it ruin our quality of life. You have a chance to overcome this challenge and set the stage for a thriving future imbued with health and happiness, so make sure you use these tips to banish sarcopenia from your life.

CHAPTER TWELVE

Nutrition's Role in Sarcopenia

Dietitians can take a proactive stance in recommending ways to prevent patients' loss of muscle mass.

Approximately 45% of older adults in the United States are affected by sarcopenia, a number that will continue to increase as the population ages. Sarcopenia, the Greek term meaning "poverty of the flesh," is the progressive loss of muscle mass, function, quality, and strength driven by the aging process. This loss of muscle mass often leads to diminished strength and decreased activity levels and can contribute to mobility issues, osteoporosis, falls and fractures, frailty, and loss of physical function and independence.

This chapter provides general information about this condition to help nutrition professionals recognize ways to assist patients in preventing sarcopenia.

Sarcopenia Stats

It's estimated that sarcopenia affects 30% of people over the age of 60 and more than 50% of those over the age of 80.3 Between the ages of 30 and 60, the average adult will gain 1 lb of weight and lose 1/2 lb of muscle yearly, a total gain of 30 lbs of fat and a loss of 15 lbs of muscle. After the age of 70, muscle loss accelerates to 15% per decade. People who are obese and also have sarcopenia (sarcopenic obesity) seem to have worse outcomes than those who aren't obese. And older adults who must be on bed rest can experience dramatic physical declines due to rapid loss of both muscle mass and strength.

Estimates indicate that 20% of older adults in the United States are functionally disabled, and the risk of disability is 1.5 to 4.6 times higher in older adults with sarcopenia than in those of the same age with normal muscle. Pathological sarcopenia is associated with a very high rate of disability. The weakness that accompanies sarcopenia can dramatically increase the risk of falls for older adults, and one-half of all accidental deaths among people over the age of 65 are related to falls. There's even some evidence that sarcopenia is related to metabolic problems, including insulin resistance, type 2 diabetes, and obesity.

The economic burden of related healthcare expenditures for sarcopenia in the United States is estimated to be $18.5 billion annually (or $900 per person per year). The cost of treating men with sarcopenia is $10.8 billion, while the cost of treating women is $7.7 billion. The greater decline in men's muscle mass is attributed to hormonal factors, including a decrease in growth hormone and testosterone levels. Janssen and colleagues estimated that a reduction of sarcopenia of just 10% would save $1.1 billion in healthcare costs.

Factors that accelerate an older adult's loss of muscle mass include decreased physical activity, testosterone and growth hormone deficiency, possibly mild cytokine excess, and the stress response. Physiological anorexia decreased caloric intake, and weight loss is all related to aging which, in turn, is associated with a decline in muscle mass and increased mortality. On average, older adults consume fewer calories and protein than younger adults. While the exact cause of the decreased intake is unclear, several theories have been advanced, including lower muscle mass resulting in lower physiological nutrient needs.

Risk factors for altered nutritional status include the following:

- Sensory changes in the ability to taste food;

- Refusal to consume meals related to restrictive therapeutic diets;

- Decreased ability to eat independently related to physical and/or cognitive decline;

- Insufficient availability of food or fluids;

- Environmental factors such as dining room atmosphere;

- Decline in instrumental activities of daily living (eg, food procurement and preparation);

- Adverse consequences of medications;

- Depression or social isolation due to the loss of a spouse or friends;

- Gastrointestinal disorders such as gastroesophageal reflux disease, chronic diarrhea, or constipation; and diseases such as Parkinson's, advanced lung or heart disease, or repetitive movement disorders (eg, pacing, wandering, rocking).

Nutrition Screening

Early screening to identify individuals at nutritional risk for unintended weight loss and undernutrition or malnutrition is essential. Nutrition professionals, physicians, healthcare facilities, and agencies should use a validated nutrition screening tool. The Mini Nutrition Assessment Short Form (MNA-SF) has been validated in both the community and healthcare settings specifically for adults over the age of 65.

The MNA-SF focuses on six variables that together identify malnutrition in older adults. The first three variables evaluate indicators of past nutrition status (weight loss), present nutrition status (BMI or calf circumference), and potential future nutrition problems (appetite). The last three variables assess important age-related factors that negatively impact nutrition in the elderly (disease, dementia or depression, and immobility). Low MNA-SF scores correlate with a decline in functional ability, cognitive impairment, and increased frailty in older adults.

The MNA-SF screening can be completed in approximately five minutes and is a stand-alone tool to identify malnourished older adults.

Other validated screening tools include the Malnutrition Screening Tool and the Malnutrition Universal Screening Tool. However, these tools aren't widely used in this country.

Nutrition Care Process

If the nutrition screening process determines an individual is at high risk for unintended weight loss, undernutrition, or malnutrition, a referral should be made to an RD. The RD should follow the Academy of Nutrition and Dietetics (the Academy) Standardized Nutrition Care Process of assessment, diagnosis, intervention, and monitoring/evaluation.

A comprehensive nutrition assessment includes a review of the nutrition screening tool, the medical record, and an interview with the individual patient or resident. The Subjective Global Assessment is a validated nutrition assessment tool. However, this isn't widely used in the United States.

Because there are few validated comprehensive nutrition assessment tools available, the assessment should include some basic information, such as the following:

- Preadmission illness, medical history, diagnosis, and recent changes in condition;

- Risk factors or signs or symptoms of undernutrition, malnutrition, dehydration, unintended weight loss, and pressure ulcers;

- Height, current weight, usual body weight, weight history, and significant changes in weight (greater than 5% in 30 days or greater than 10% in 180 days);

- Current food and fluid intake adequacy compared with calculated nutritional needs;

- Eating ability (able to feed self, requires assistance, needs total assistance);

- Interview with the individual and/or family or staff for food preferences and tolerances;

- Medications that may affect food or fluid intake or tolerance (eg, food-medication interactions);

- Other factors that may impact nutritional status (eg, chewing/swallowing ability, gastrointestinal problems, depression);

- Current nutrition interventions (eg, food or dining interventions, oral nutritional supplements); and monitoring and evaluating nutritional status and outcomes.

In addition to these factors, a nutrition-focused physical examination should include an inspection of the body to determine information regarding the individual's nutritional status. Visual assessment of overall appearance can help identify underweight or cachexia, muscle wasting, abdominal distention, edema, and/or weakness in the extremities, all of which may indicate protein-energy malnutrition. The oral examination may reveal issues with chewing and/or swallowing. Skin examinations help assess for the presence of ulcers, skin tears, bruises, turgor, or dryness.

Biochemical data analysis may help clinicians evaluate overall health issues; however, care must be taken when interpreting lab values for use as nutritional markers. Although markers of protein status, such as albumin and prealbumin, may assist the clinician to establish the overall prognosis and severity of illness, they aren't accurate markers of protein or nutritional status.

It's important to review laboratory values for anemia and/or dehydration. When anemia is present, the blood has reduced oxygen-carrying capacity, which can lead to various side effects and negative consequences, such as lower endurance, impaired temperature regulation, decreased immune function, increased rates of infection, impaired cognitive functioning/memory, and possibly increased mortality in older adults. Dehydration can have serious consequences for older adults, including decreased functional ability, predisposition to falls and infections, fluid and electrolyte imbalances, disorientation, and even death.

The care plan should be developed based on the assessment and the risk factors identified, and the goals should be measurable. Interventions should be individualized, aggressive, and revised as often as needed based on responses, outcomes, and needs.

Key Nutrition Recommendations

In 2008, the Society for Sarcopenia, Cachexia, and Wasting convened an expert panel to develop nutritional recommendations for sarcopenia prevention and management. For preventing and treating this condition, protein and energy intake are key components, along with both resistance and aerobic exercise.

Protein

Older adults historically are at risk of protein intake below the Recommended Dietary Allowance (RDA) for healthy adults (0.8 g/kg/day). Older adults fail to ingest the highest acceptable macronutrient distribution for the protein of 35% of energy intake. One study of adults over the age of 50 noted that 27% to 41% of women and 15% to 38% of men consumed less than the RDA for protein.

Several studies illustrate the correlation between protein ingestion and muscle mass. Ingestion of protein-deficient meals fails to stimulate protein synthesis because the availability of blood amino acids isn't increased. The prime responsibility of essential amino acids in the regulation of protein synthesis, and leucine seems to be the most beneficial amino acid. Leucine is a precursor for protein synthesis and stimulates the specific intracellular pathway associated with muscle protein synthesis.

Metabolic changes in older adults result in the production of less muscle protein than for younger adults who consume the same amount of dietary protein.

Studies indicate that an amino acid mixture of 30 g per meal produced protein synthesis similar to younger people. The expert panel recommended a total protein intake of 1 to 1.5 g/kg/day with equal amounts of protein consumed at breakfast, lunch, and dinner.24 This would be equivalent to 69 to 102 g/day for a person weighing 150 lbs (23 to 34 g per meal).

Supplementing the diet with whey protein is beneficial because whey protein delivers the correct amino acids in proportion to the ratio of skeletal muscle. Whey protein supplementation stimulates an important mechanism that preserves muscle mass by creating and maintaining a high concentration of essential amino acids in the blood. When protein supplementation (15 to 20 g) increased the muscle-strengthening effects of resistance exercise. Creatine may improve the effects of exercise on sarcopenic individuals, but additional studies are recommended.

Muscles are made of protein and most mature adults don't get enough. Some studies suggest that the daily protein requirement for people over sixty years is greater than that of younger people. All of the studies of sarcopenia relate inadequate protein intake with rapid loss of muscle mass.

There's no set amount of protein that fits every person; however, noticeable loss in muscle mass is an indication that you're not getting enough. Increase in protein intake in tandem with RT has been proven effective in restoring muscle mass and strength. Please note that a protein-rich diet is contraindicated for people with impaired kidney function.

Part of the challenge with getting enough protein as we age is the body's increasing inability to process it. Proteins should come from variety of sources, not just animal meat (which is acidic). Other foods with significant protein include:

- nuts
- seeds
- quinoa
- kefir
- beans
- eggs
- tofu and tempeh
- hemp
- cheese
- teff
- avocado.

Vitamin D

Vitamin D deficiency is the most prevalent nutritional deficiency for older adults regardless of race or ethnicity. Levels of 25-hydroxyvitamin D [25(OH)] decreases with age. Depleted vitamin D levels are associated with low muscle strength. Supplementation of vitamin D in individuals with low levels increases muscle strength. 25(OH) vitamin D levels should be measured in all sarcopenic individuals and vitamin D supplementation in doses sufficient to increase levels above 100 nmol/L should be given as an adjunctive therapy. Dosages of 50,000 IU of vitamins D2 or D3 per week are acceptable.

Clinical Strategy

Tips for Adding Protein
- Add cheese to vegetables, salads, potatoes, rice, noodles, and casseroles.

- Add hard-cooked eggs to salads.

- Consider Greek yogurt alone or add to fruit and cereal.

- Supplement diet with high-protein bars or a fruit smoothie made with milk or yogurt.

- Add peanut butter to sandwiches, toast, crackers, or muffins or use as a dip for vegetables and fruit.

- Add powdered milk to cream soups, mashed potatoes, casseroles, puddings, and milk-based desserts.

- Add a scoop of powdered milk, whey protein, or powdered commercial supplement mix to each cup of regular milk (2 cups) daily. These also can be added into hot cereal.

- Select commercial supplements with high-quality protein.

- Add nuts, seeds, or wheat germ to casseroles, breads, muffins, pancakes, and cookies, or use nuts, seeds, or wheat germ to top fruit, cereal, ice cream, and yogurt or in place of breadcrumbs.

- Add beans (eg, navy, kidney, pinto, black) and lentils to soups, casseroles, or salads.

Physical Activity

Nearly all older adults can benefit from resistance and strength training to increase muscle strength, improve functional ability, or prevent further decline. There are four components of physical activity that are important for a well- balanced exercise plan. Resistance exercise, in particular, has been shown to decrease frailty and improve muscle strength in very elderly adults. Exercise is recommended on most days of the week, but a minimum of three times per week is suggested to slow muscle loss and prevent sarcopenia.

Overall, endurance exercises improve the cardiovascular and circulatory systems (low-impact exercises). Strength training reduces sarcopenia, builds muscle, and possibly prevents osteoporosis. Alone and in combination with nutritional supplementation, strength training increases strength and functional capacity. Balance exercises such as tai chi or something as simple as standing on one leg with eyes closed (possibly while holding onto a stationary object) can help prevent falls. And flexibility exercises such as yoga or stretching can help older adults recover from or prevent injuries or falls.

Nutrition and exercise together have a synergistic effect that helps combat malnutrition, increases strength, and promotes well-being. Encourage physical activity and suggest age- and ability-appropriate exercises, including walking and strength training. Refer patients to a physical therapist to assess a range of motion, strength, and endurance and to determine the need for assistive devices such as canes, walkers, grab bars, or shower chairs. Determine whether an elder can benefit from continued physical therapy, occupational therapy, or strength training and refer to social services for a home environment assessment as appropriate.

Hormone and Drug Therapies

Testosterone therapy for men with low testosterone levels has been linked to the increased muscle mass; however, it hasn't been associated with improved functional performance or a reduction in mortality. In addition, cardiac complications and prostate cancer are potential risks of testosterone therapy. More research is needed to determine whether therapy is safe relative to the benefits it produces.

Growth hormone hasn't been shown to reverse sarcopenic symptoms in older adults, and it may create profound side effects. Angiotensin-converting enzyme inhibitors show some promise in treating muscle atrophy and reducing inflammation. Selective androgen receptor modulators are a promising new class of drugs that may act similarly to testosterone without the negative side effects.

Prevention Is Key

It's more effective to adopt strategies designed to prevent or slow the progression of sarcopenia than it is to try to treat the condition in elderly patients. Recommending dietary modifications, nutritional supplements, exercise, and possibly hormone replacement therapy can be appropriate steps to combat muscle deterioration. Maximizing muscle mass can improve older adults' functionality, strength, endurance, and general health.

CHAPTER THIRTEEN

What is good for Sarcopenia?

By trying the following methods, you can fight sarcopenia, as well as strengthening your muscles, you can be protected from muscle loss.

Epsom Salt Bath

The Epsom salt, also known as magnesium sulfate, is a compound made of magnesium sulfur and oxygen that is completely different from the table salt. Used as a bath salt. Epsom salt bath strengthens and relaxes your muscles and provides a general relief. To prepare the bath, fill a standard bath tub with warm water, add about 2 cups of Epsom salt and let it melt. Then, lie in that water for 15 minutes.

Massage

Massage on the body with coconut oil, olive oil, and mustard oil eases the blood flow by relaxing the muscles. With the acceleration of the bloodstream, vitamins, and minerals that feed muscles like protein, iron, and magnesium, reach the muscles more easily and strengthen the muscles.

Water

Dehydration is a factor that weakens the muscles in the person. At least 2 liters of water consumption during the day muscle tension can be prevented as well as muscles can be strengthened.

Acupressure

Acupressure is a method similar to acupuncture. Pressure is applied to the acupuncture areas and it is aimed to reduce the pain in that area. Although acupressure is mainly used to relieve pain, it also accelerates the bloodstream and helps to strengthen muscles.

Foods with Vitamin D

Vitamin D supplements can be used to prevent muscle weakness and loss. Muscles can also be strengthened by sunbathing for 10 minutes in the morning. Salmon, fish, milk, orange juice, and spinach are rich in vitamin D also very beneficial.

Does Sarcopenia kill? How long patients do live?

In cases where sarcopenia progresses, is not diagnosed and treated early, the disease can have fatal consequences. When the diagnosis and treatment of the disease are delayed, it is only possible to extend the life span of the patients at least a few years by treatment methods such as physical therapy, exercise, and proper nutrition.

What would Sarcopenia Patients eat?

A diet rich in vitamin D, magnesium, and calcium can be effective in the treatment of muscle loss.

- Protein: Increases muscle growth by enhancing muscle tissue. Muscle growth can be achieved by eating lean meat, fish, eggs, and soy.

- Vitamin D: Vitamin D supplements can help to stop this process because vitamin D deficiency is an important cause of muscle loss.

- Omega 3: 2 grams of fish oil supplement daily with regular resistance training is especially effective in the treatment of muscle loss in the elderly. This is thought to be due to the anti-inflammatory properties of Omega 3 fatty acids.

- Mediterranean type diet: A Mediterranean type diet including fish, olive oil, and dark green leafy vegetables can provide positive results for sarcopenia treatment.

- Keratin: Many scientific studies are suggesting that keratin administration with regular exercise helps muscle growth. However, keratin intake alone is not sufficient.

Suggestions to Sarcopenia Patients

- Remember that stress accelerates the process of sarcopenia and try to keep your morale as high as possible.

- Take care to consume foods that strengthen muscles such as bananas, honey, and yogurt.

- Believe in the strength of exercise and do the exercises that your physiotherapist recommends daily.

- Do not smoke or drink alcohol.

- Limit caffeine consumption as much as possible.

- Regulate your sleep.

Strategies to Prevent Age-Related Muscle Loss

Sarcopenia, the loss of skeletal muscle mass and strength, is a major problem as people age. It can lead to disability, osteoporosis, falls, hospital stays, and even death. Wondering how to prevent sarcopenia? Taking a few natural steps now can improve muscle health and help maintain autonomy and well-being into old age.

Start with an Understanding of Causes

Two of the most preventable and treatable factors that contribute to sarcopenia are lack of exercise and poor nutrition.

Older adults spend most of their waking hours engaged in sedentary activities. Inactivity accelerates muscle breakdown and dysfunction, often leading to a vicious cycle of muscle loss, injury, and inefficient repair, causing elderly people to become increasingly sedentary over time.

Many older Americans fail to consume the current recommended dietary allowance (RDA) of protein, which may not even be high enough for their needs, Older people require more protein than younger people to stimulate the same amount of muscle growth.,

Diagnosing Sarcopenia

Sarcopenia is diagnosed using the criteria of low muscle mass and low muscle function (either low strength and/or low physical performance)., The three most important tests for diagnosing sarcopenia are appendicular lean body mass, grip strength, and gait speed.

Appendicular skeletal muscle mass. Imaging techniques used for estimating muscle mass include computed tomography (CT scan), magnetic resonance imaging (MRI), and dual-energy X-ray absorptiometry (DXA). CT and MRI are gold standard methods but are rarely used because of their high cost, limited access, and concerns about radiation exposure. DXA is the method most often used in research because it is less expensive and exposes the patient to minimal radiation.

A practical alternative for measuring muscle mass, and one you can even use on your own at home, is bioelectrical impedance analysis (BIA). When used in clinics, BIA has been found to correlate well with body imaging techniques like MRI and is considered by experts to be an appropriate alternative to DXA in the diagnosis of sarcopenia.,

Home BIA machines are commonly called "body fat scales" or "body composition analyzers." Most devices display some measurement of muscle mass, such as muscle mass percentage or muscle mass in weight.

Handgrip strength is currently the most popular, well-studied, and best-accepted way of assessing muscle strength and diagnosing sarcopenia.

Grip strength accurately measures general upper body strength and reflects overall strength, lower-limb strength, and performance., It is positively and significantly associated with cognition, functional status, mobility, cardiovascular disease, and death. Even in middle-aged people, grip strength is an accurate and consistent predictor of all causes of death.,

To measure handgrip strength, a person squeezes a dynamometer as hard as they can three times, with a one-minute rest between measurements. The highest value of <30 kg for men or <20 kg for women is the cut-off for diagnosing sarcopenia. These values identify weaknesses associated with limitations in mobility.

Dynamometers are available for personal purchase but are fairly expensive. If you don't have access to your own, many doctor's offices, health clinics, and fitness centers have dynamometers available for assessing strength.

Gait speed is a simple, well-documented marker of physical performance. To assess gait speed, mark off a six-meter course. Measure the time, in seconds, it takes to complete the walk at your usual pace. Walking aids are allowed.

Gait speed <0.8 meters per second denotes mobility impairment. Gait speed ≤0.8 m/s is the recommended cut-off value in the diagnosis of sarcopenia and predicts subsequent disability, falls, cognitive decline, institutionalization, and mortality.

CONCLUSION

Sarcopenia remains an important clinical problem that impacts millions of older adults. Causes of this condition include declines in hormones and numbers of neuromuscular junctions, increased inflammation, declines in inactivity, and inadequate nutrition. There are a lot of conditions correlated with sarcopenias like obesity, diabetes, and reduced account of Vitamin D. It has been proposed that excess energy intake, physical inactivity, low-grade inflammation, insulin resistance, and changes in hormonal homeostasis may result in the development of sarcopenic obesity. Sarcopenia is highly correlated with frailty and risk of falls in the elderly, it also represents an important risk factor for disability and mortality. Therefore, sarcopenia has a greater effect on survival. Accordingly, to this evidence, it should be important to prevent or postpone as much as possible the onset of sarcopenia among older people, to enhance survival, and to reduce the demand for long-term care. Interventions for sarcopenia continue to be developed, and the interest in sarcopenia must be increased, in particular by analyzing the effect of exercise and nutritional interventions.

HOW TO FIGHT MUSCLE LOSS AS YOU AGE?

As you've learned throughout this book, sarcopenia is a serious condition that affects countless older adults, robbing them of their strength, independence, and quality of life. The gradual loss of muscle mass and function may seem inevitable, but you now know that there are powerful strategies you can employ to fight back against this age-related decline.

The causes of sarcopenia are complex and multifaceted, ranging from hormonal changes and neurological factors to chronic inflammation and sedentary lifestyles. You've discovered that as you age, your body produces less testosterone, growth hormone, and insulin-like growth factor-1 (IGF-1), all of which play crucial roles in maintaining muscle mass.

Additionally, the number of neuromuscular junctions declines, impairing the connection between your nerves and muscles.

Inflammation, a common feature of aging, also contributes to sarcopenia by breaking down muscle tissue and inhibiting muscle regeneration. You've learned that conditions like obesity and diabetes can exacerbate this inflammation, creating a vicious cycle that accelerates muscle loss.

The combination of sarcopenia and obesity, known as sarcopenic obesity, poses a particularly significant threat to your health and mobility.

Here, you've discovered the importance of staying physically active and engaging in regular resistance training to combat sarcopenia. By challenging your muscles with weights or bodyweight exercises, you stimulate the growth of new muscle fibers and maintain the ones you already have.

Remember, it's never too late to start, and even small amounts of exercise can make a big difference.

Nutrition also plays a vital role in fighting sarcopenia. You've learned about the importance of consuming adequate protein, particularly from high-quality sources like lean meats, fish, eggs, and legumes.

Aim to distribute your protein intake evenly throughout the day, as your body can only use a certain amount at a time for muscle synthesis.

Don't forget about the role of vitamin D, which helps maintain muscle strength and function. Ensure you're getting enough through sunlight exposure, fortified foods, or supplements if necessary.

Key Takeaways:

- Sarcopenia is a multifaceted condition caused by hormonal changes, neurological factors, inflammation, inactivity, and poor nutrition.

- Engaging in regular resistance training is crucial for maintaining muscle mass and strength as you age.

- Consuming adequate protein, evenly distributed throughout the day, supports muscle health.

- Ensuring enough vitamin D intake helps maintain muscle function.

- Staying active and addressing underlying conditions like obesity and diabetes can help combat sarcopenia.

Sarcopenia can be a serious condition, leading to many additional physical and mental health problems. If you feel like you may be losing muscles and are not as strong as you used to be, exercise and a healthy, protein-rich diet can help you build up strength. Some people may benefit from taking hormones such as testosterone or human growth hormone. If you think you may have sarcopenia, talk to your doctor to come up with a treatment plan that can work well for your needs.

As you start on your path to fight sarcopenia, remember that consistency is key. Making exercise and healthy nutrition a part of your daily routine will yield the best results over time. Embrace the power of small, incremental changes, and celebrate the progress you make along the way.

REFERENCES

1. Goldspink DF. Aging and activity: their effects on the functional reserve capacities of the heart and vascular smooth and skeletal muscles. Ergonomics. 2007;48(11– 14):1334–51.

2. Frontera WR, Ochala J. Skeletal Muscle: A Brief Review of Structure and Function. Calcif Tissue Int [Internet]. 2014; Available from: http://link.springer.com/10.1007/s00223-014-9915-y

3. Mitchell WK, Williams J, Atherton P, Larvin M, Lund J, Narici M. Sarcopenia, dynapenia, and the impact of advancing age on human skeletal muscle size and strength; a quantitative review. Front Physiol. 2012;3 JUL(July):1–18.

4. Guralnik JM, Ferrucci L, Simonsick EM, Salive ME, Wallace RB. Lower-extremity function in persons over the age of 70 years is a predictor of subsequent disability. N Engl J Med. 1995;332(9):556–61.

5. Burton L a., Sumukadas D. Optimal management of sarcopenia. Clin Interv Aging. 2010;5:217-28.

6. Aagaard P, Suetta C, Caserotti P, Magnusson SP, Kjær M. Role of the nervous system in sarcopenia and muscle atrophy with aging: Strength training as a countermeasure. Scand J Med Sci Sport. 2010;20(1):49-64.

7. Cruz-Jentoft AJ, Baeyens JP, Bauer JM, Boirie Y, Cederholm T, Landi F, et al. Sarcopenia: European consensus on definition and diagnosis. Age Ageing. 2010;39(4):412-23.

8. Cooper R, Kuh D, Cooper C, Gale CR, Lawlor D a., Matthews F, et al. Objective measures of physical capability and subsequent health: A systematic review. Age Ageing. 2011;40(1):14-23.

9. Rizzoli R, Reginster J, Arnal J, Bautmans I. Quality of Life in Sarcopenia and Frailty. Calcif Tissue Int. 2014;93(2):101-20.

10. Janssen I, Shepard DS, Katzmarzyk PT, Roubenoff R. The healthcare costs of sarcopenia in the United States. J Am Geriatr Soc. 2004;52(1):80-5.

11. Baumgartner RN, Koehler KM, Gallagher D, Romero L, Heymsfield SB, Ross RR, et al. Epidemiology of sarcopenia among the elderly in New Mexico. Am J Epidemiol. 1998;147(8):755-63.

12. Melton LJ, Khosla S, Crowson CS, Michael K, Connor O, Fallon WMO, et al. Epidemiology of Sarcopenia. J Am Geriatr Soc. 2000;48:625-30.

13. Janssen I, Heymsfield SB, Ross R. Low relative skeletal muscle mass (sarcopenia) is Associated with Functional Impairment and Physical Disability. Am Geriatr Soc. 2002;50:889-96.

14. Tankó LB, Movsesyan L, Mouritzen U, Christiansen C, Svendsen OL. Appendicular lean tissue mass and the prevalence of sarcopenia among healthy women. Metabolism. 2002;51(1):69-74.

15. Iannuzzi-Sucich M, Prestwood KM, Kenny AM. Prevalence of sarcopenia and predictors of skeletal muscle mass in healthy, older men and women. J Gerontol A Biol Sci Med Sci. 2002;57(12):M772-7.

16. Rolland Y, Dupuy C, Abellan van Kan G, Gillette S, Vellas B. Treatment Strategies for Sarcopenia and Frailty. Vol. 95, Medical Clinics of North America. 2011. p. 427- 38.

17. Gillette-Guyonnet S, Nourhashemi F, Andrieu S, Cantet C, Albarède JL, Vellas B, et al. Body composition in French women 75+ years of age: The EPIDOS study. Mech Ageing Dev. 2003;124(3):311-6.

18. Newman AB, Kupelian V, Visser M, Simonsick E, Goodpaster B, Nevitt M, et al. Sarcopenia: Alternative Definitions and Associations with LowerExtremity Function. J Am Geriatr Soc. 2003;51:1602-9.

19. Castillo EM, Goodman-Gruen D, Kritz-Silverstein D, Morton DJ, Wingard DL, Barrett-Connor E. Sarcopenia in elderly men and women: The Rancho Bernardo study. Am J

Prev Med. 2003;25(3):226-31.

20. Sayer AA, Dennison EM, Syddall HE, Jameson K, Martin HJ, Cooper C. The developmental origins of sarcopenia: using peripheral quantitative computed tomography to assess muscle size in older people. J Gerontol A Biol Sci Med Sci. 2008;63(8):835-40.

21. Campbell WW, Trappe T a, Wolfe RR, Evans WJ. The recommended dietary allowance for protein may not be adequate for older people to maintain skeletal muscle. J Gerontol A Biol Sci Med Sci. 2001;56(6):M373-80.

22. Burd N a, Gorissen SH, van Loon LJC. Anabolic resistance of muscle protein synthesis with aging. Exerc Sport Sci Rev. 2013;41(3):169-73

23. Reid KF, Pasha E, Doros G, Clark DJ, Patten C, Phillips EM, et al. The longitudinal decline of lower extremity muscle power in healthy and mobility-limited older adults: Influence of muscle mass, strength, composition, neuromuscular activation, and single fiber contractile properties. Eur J Appl Physiol. 2014;114(1):29-39.

24. Malafarina V, Uriz-Otano F, Iniesta R, Gil-Guerrero L. Effectiveness of Nutritional Supplementation on Muscle Mass in Treatment of Sarcopenia in Old Age: A Systematic Review. J Am Med Dir Assoc. 2013;14(1):10- 7.

25. Goldspink DF. Aging and activity: their effects on the functional reserve capacities of the heart and vascular smooth and skeletal muscles. Ergonomics. 2007;48(11- 14):1334-51.

26. Hayes KC, Wolfe DL, Trujillo S a, Burkell J a. On the interaction of disability and aging: Accelerated degradation models and their influence on projections of future care needs and costs for personal injury litigation. Disabil Rehabil. 2010;32(5):424–8.

27. Evans WJ. Skeletal muscle loss: Cachexia, sarcopenia, and inactivity. Am J Clin Nutr. 2010;91(4):1123–7.

28. Smith L, Gardner B, Fisher a., Hamer M. Patterns and correlates of physical activity behavior over 10 years in older adults: prospective analyses from the English Longitudinal Study of Ageing. BMJ Open. 2015;5(4):1-5.

29. Mitchell WK, Williams J, Atherton P, Larvin M, Lund J, Narici M. Sarcopenia, dynapenia, and the impact of advancing age on human skeletal muscle size and strength; a quantitative review. Front Physiol. 2012;3 JUL(July):1–18.

30. Balagopal P, Schimke JC, Ades P, Adey D, Nair KS. Age effect on transcript levels and synthesis rate of muscle MHC and response to resistance exercise. Am J Physiol Endocrinol Metab. 2001;280(2):E203– 8.

31. Burton L a., Sumukadas D. Optimal management of sarcopenia. Clin Interv Aging. 2010;5:217–28.

32. Aagaard P, Suetta C, Caserotti P, Magnusson SP, Kjær M. Role of the nervous system in sarcopenia and muscle atrophy with aging: Strength training as a countermeasure. Scand J Med Sci Sport. 2010;20(1):49–64.

33. Morley JE, Abbatecola AM, Argiles JM, Baracos V, Bauer J,

Bhasin S, et al.

34. Sarcopenia With Limited Mobility: An International Consensus. J Am Med Dir Assoc. 2011;12(6):403–9.

35. Rosenberg IH. Sarcopenia: Origins and Clinical Relevance. Am Soc Nutr Sci. 1997;127(May):990–1.

36. Baumgartner RN, Koehler KM, Gallagher D, Romero L, Heymsfield SB, Ross RR, et al. Epidemiology of sarcopenia among the elderly in New Mexico. Am J Epidemiol. 1998;147(8):755–63.

37. Janssen I, Heymsfield SB, Ross R. Low relative skeletal muscle mass (sarcopenia) is Associated with Functional Impairment and Physical Disability. Am Geriatr Soc. 2002;50:889–96.

38. Harris T. Muscle mass and strength: relation to function in population studies. J Nutr. 1997;127(5 Suppl):1004S–1006S.

39. Cruz-Jentoft AJ, Baeyens JP, Bauer JM, Boirie Y, Cederholm T, Landi F, et al.

40. Sarcopenia: European consensus on definition and diagnosis. Age Ageing. 2010;39(4):412–23.

41. Chen LK, Liu LK, Woo J, Assantachai P, Auyeung TW, Bahyah KS, et al. Sarcopenia in Asia: Consensus report of the Asian working group for sarcopenia. J Am Med Dir Assoc [Internet]. Elsevier Ltd; 2014;15(2):95–101. Available from: http://dx.doi.org/10.1016/j.jamda.2013.11.025

42. Fielding R a., Vellas B, Evans WJ, Bhasin S, Morley JE, Newman AB, et al.

43. Sarcopenia: An Undiagnosed Condition in Older Adults. Current Consensus Definition: Prevalence, Etiology, and Consequences. International Working Group on Sarcopenia. J Am Med Dir Assoc. Elsevier Ltd; 2011;12(4):249–56. Available from: http://dx.doi.org/10.1016/j.jamda.2011.01.003

44. Studenski S a., Peters KW, Alley DE, Cawthon PM, McLean RR, Harris TB, et al. The FNIH sarcopenia project: Rationale, study description, conference recommendations, and final estimates. Journals Gerontol - Ser A Biol Sci Med Sci. 2014;69 A(5):547–58.

45. Dam TT, Peters KW, Fragala M, Cawthon PM, Harris TB, McLean R, et al. An evidence-based comparison of operational criteria for the presence of sarcopenia. Journals Gerontol - Ser A Biol Sci Med Sci. 2014;69 A(5):584–90.

46. Melton LJ, Khosla S, Crowson CS, Michael K, Connor O, Fallon WMO, et al. Epidemiology of Sarcopenia. J Am Geriatr Soc. 2000;48:625–30.

47. Morley JE, Baumgartner RN, Roubenoff R, Mayer J, Nair KS. Sarcopenia. J Lab Clin Med. 2001;137(4):231–43.

48. Tankó LB, Movsesyan L, Mouritzen U, Christiansen C, Svendsen OL. Appendicular lean tissue mass and the prevalence of sarcopenia among healthy women. Metabolism. 2002;51(1):69–74.

49. Iannuzzi-Sucich M, Prestwood KM, Kenny AM. Prevalence of sarcopenia and predictors of skeletal muscle mass in healthy, older men and women. J Gerontol A Biol Sci Med Sci. 2002;57(12):M772–7.

50. Gillette-Guyonnet S, Nourhashemi F, Andrieu S, Cantet C, Albarède JL, Vellas B, et al. Body composition in French women 75+ years of age: The EPIDOS study. Mech Ageing Dev. 2003;124(3):311–6.

51. Newman AB, Kupelian V, Visser M, Simonsick E, Goodpaster B, Nevitt M, et al.

52. Sarcopenia: Alternative Definitions and Associations with Lower Extremity Function. J Am Geriatr Soc. 2003;51:1602–9.

53. Castillo EM, Goodman-Gruen D, Kritz-Silverstein D, Morton DJ, Wingard DL, Barrett-Connor E. Sarcopenia in elderly men and women: The Rancho Bernardo study. Am J Prev Med. 2003;25(3):226–31.

54. Janssen I, Baumgartner RN, Ross R, Rosenberg IH, Roubenoff R. Skeletal Muscle Cutpoints Associated with Elevated Physical Disability Risk in Older Men and Women. Am J Epidemiol. 2004;159(4):413–21.

55. Beaudart C, Reginster J, Slomian J, Buckinx F, Locquet M, Bruyère O. Prevalence of sarcopenia: the impact of different diagnostic cut-off limits. 2014;14(4):425–31.

56. Lau EMC, Lynn HSH, Woo JW, Kwok TCY, Melton LJ. Prevalence of and risk factors for sarcopenia in elderly Chi-

nese men and women. J Gerontol A Biol Sci Med Sci. 2005;60(2):213-6.

57. Chien MY, Huang TY, Wu YT. Prevalence of sarcopenia estimated using a bioelectrical impedance analysis prediction equation in community-dwelling elderly people in Taiwan. J Am Geriatr Soc. 2008;56:1710-5.

58. Janssen I, Shepard DS, Katzmarzyk PT, Roubenoff R. The healthcare costs of sarcopenia in the United States. J Am Geriatr Soc. 2004;52(1):80-5.

59. Malafarina V, Úriz-Otano F, Iniesta R, Gil-Guerrero L. Sarcopenia in the elderly: Diagnosis, physiopathology, and treatment. Maturitas. 2012;71(2):109-14.

60. Short KR, Nair KS. The effect of age on protein metabolism. Curr Opin Clin Nutr Metab Care. 2000;3(1):39-44.

61. Rizzoli R, Reginster J, Arnal J, Bautmans I. Quality of Life in Sarcopenia and Frailty. Calcif Tissue Int. 2014;93(2):101-20.

62. Kwan Ping. Sarcopenia, a neurogenic syndrome? J Aging Res. 2013;2013. Available from:http://dx.doi.org/10.1155/2013/791679

63. Guralnik JM, Ferrucci L, Simonsick EM, Salive ME, Wallace RB. Lower-extremity function in persons over the age of 70 years is a predictor of subsequent disability. N Engl J Med. 1995;332(9):556-61.

64. Cooper R, Kuh D, Cooper C, Gale CR, Lawlor D a.,

Matthews F, et al. Objective measures of physical capability and subsequent health: A systematic review. Age Ageing. 2011;40(1):14–23.

65. Lauretani F, Russo CR, Bandinelli S, Bartali B, Cavazzini C, Di Iorio A, et al. Age-associated changes in skeletal muscles and their effect on mobility: an operational diagnosis of sarcopenia. J Appl Physiol. 2003;95(5):1851–60.

66. Short KR, Vittone JL, Bigelow ML, Proctor DN, Rizza R a., Coenen-Schimke JM, et al. Impact of Aerobic Exercise Training on Age-Related Changes in Insulin Sensitivity and Muscle Oxidative Capacity. Diabetes. 2003;52(8):1888–96.

67. Cox JH, Cortright RN, Dohm GL, Houmard J a. Effect of aging on response to exercise training in humans: skeletal muscle GLUT-4 and insulin sensitivity. J Appl Physiol. 1999;86(6):2019–25.

68. Johnson ML, Lanza IR, Short DK, Asmann YW, Nair KS. Chronically endurancetrained individuals preserve skeletal muscle mitochondrial gene expression with age but differences within age groups remain. Physiol Rep. 2014;2(12):e12239–e12239. Available from: http://physreports.physiology.org/cgi/doi/10.14814/phy2.12239

69. Leveille SG, Guralnik JM, Ferrucci L, Langlois J a. Aging successfully until death in old age: opportunities for increasing active life expectancy. Am J Epidemiol. 1999;149(7):654–64.

70. Ferrando a a, Tipton KD, Bamman MM, Wolfe RR. Re-

sistance exercise maintains skeletal muscle protein synthesis during bed rest. J Appl Physiol. 1997;82(3):807–10.

71. Liu C, Latham NK. Progressive resistance strength training for improving physical function in older adults. Cochrane Database Syst Rev. 2009;29(6):997–1003.

72. Szulc P, Munoz F, Marchand F, Chapurlat R, Delmas PD. Rapid loss of appendicular skeletal muscle mass is associated with higher all-cause mortality in older men: The prospective MINOS study. Am J Clin Nutr. 2010;91(5):1227–36.

73. Kryger a. I, Andersen JL. Resistance training in the oldest old: Consequences for muscle strength, fiber types, fiber size, and MHC isoforms. Scand J Med Sci Sport. 2007;17(4):422–30.

74. Fiatarone M a, Marks EC, Ryan ND, Meredith CN, Lipsitz L a, Evans WJ. Highintensity strength training in nonagenarians. Effects on skeletal muscle. Vol. 263, JAMA: The Journal of the American Medical Association. 1990. p. 3029–34.

75. Peterson MD, Gordon PM. Resistance exercise for the aging adult: Clinical implications and prescription guidelines. Am J Med. 2011;124(3):194–8. Available from: http://dx.doi.org/10.1016/j.amjmed.2010.08.020

76. Goodpaster BH, Chomentowski P, Ward BK, Rossi A, Glynn NW, Delmonico MJ, et al. Effects of physical activity on strength and skeletal muscle fat infiltration in older adults: a randomized controlled trial.

2008;15213:1498–503.

77. Landi F, Marzetti E, Martone AM, Bernabei R, Onder G. Exercise as a remedy for sarcopenia. Curr Opin Clin Nutr Metab Care. 2014;17(1):25–31. Available from: http://www.ncbi.nlm.nih.gov/pubmed/24310054

78. Sayer AA, Dennison EM, Syddall HE, Jameson K, Martin HJ, Cooper C. The developmental origins of sarcopenia: using peripheral quantitative computed tomography to assess muscle size in older people. J Gerontol A Biol Sci Med Sci. 2008;63(8):835–40.

79. Krogh-Madsen R, Thyfault JP, Broholm C, Mortensen OH, Olsen RH, Mounier R, et al. A 2-week reduction of ambulatory activity attenuates peripheral insulin sensitivity. J Appl Physiol. 2010;108(5):1034–40.

80. Kortebein P. Effect of 10 days of bed rest on skeletal muscle in healthy older adults. JAMA. 2009;297(16):1772–4.

81. Paddon-Jones D, Short KR, Campbell WW, Volpi E, Wolfe RR. Role of dietary protein in the sarcopenia of aging 1 – 4. Am J Clin Nutr. 2008;87:1562–6.

82. Campbell WW, Trappe T a, Wolfe RR, Evans WJ. The recommended dietary allowance for protein may not be adequate for older people to maintain skeletal muscle. J Gerontol A Biol Sci Med Sci. 2001;56(6):M373–80.

83. Deutz NEP, Bauer JM, Barazzoni R, Biolo G, Boirie Y, Bosy-Westphal A, et al. Protein intake and exercise for optimal muscle function with aging: Recommendations from

the ESPEN Expert Group. Clin Nutr. 2014;33(6):929–36. Available from: http://dx.doi.org/10.1016/j.clnu.2014.04.007

84. Burd N a, Gorissen SH, van Loon LJC. Anabolic resistance of muscle protein synthesis with aging. Exerc Sport Sci Rev. 2013;41(3):169–73. Available from: http://www.ncbi.nlm.nih.gov/pubmed/23558692

85. Smidt GL, Rogers MW. Factors contributing to the regulation and clinical assessment of muscular strength. Phys Ther. 1982;62(9):1283–90.

86. Kannus P. Isokinetic evaluation of muscular performance: implication for muscular testing and rehabilitation. Int J Sports Med. 1994;15(1):S11-8.

87. Peterson MD, Rhea MR, Sen A, Gordon PM. Resistance exercise for muscular strength in older adults: A meta-analysis. Ageing Res Rev. 2010;9(3):226–37. Available from: http://dx.doi.org/10.1016/j.arr.2010.03.004

88. Frontera WR, Hughes V a, Fielding R a, Fiatarone M a, Evans WJ, Roubenoff R. Aging of skeletal muscle: a 12-yr longitudinal study. J Appl Physiol. 2000;88(4):1321–6

89. Hughes V a, Frontera WR, Wood M, Evans WJ, Dallal GE, Roubenoff R, et al. Longitudinal muscle strength changes in older adults: influence of muscle mass, physical activity, and health. J Gerontol A Biol Sci Med Sci. 2001;56(5):B209–17.

90. Clark BC, Manini TM. Functional consequences of sarcopenia and dynapenia in the elderly. Curr Opin Clin Nutr

Metab Care. 2010;13(3):271–6.

91. Reid KF, Pasha E, Doros G, Clark DJ, Patten C, Phillips EM, et al. Longitudinal decline of lower extremity muscle power in healthy and mobility-limited older adults: Influence of muscle mass, strength, composition, neuromuscular activation, and single fiber contractile properties. Eur J Appl Physiol. 2014;114(1):29–39.

THANK YOU

Thank you for your purchase!!
If you enjoyed this book,
please consider dropping us a review on the link below:

https://www.amazon.com/review/create-review/?asin=B096TRWYWC

Your feedback goes a long way toward helping
Indie Self Publishers like our tiny business succeed.
I truly value your opinion!!

Please send an email if you have any suggestions.
Email Address: info@sliceoflife.co

I love coming up with new things that are
entertaining and full of value for you!

FIRST EDITION VOLUME 1

www.ingramcontent.com/pod-product-compliance
Lightning Source LLC
Chambersburg PA
CBHW070640220526
45466CB00001B/240